Understanding the Aspects of Nutrition for a Healthy Life

Dr. Munir A. Chandniwala

Printed in India

IndiePress

ISBN: 978-93-6045-178-3

First Printing, 2024

Indie Press

A division of Nasadiya Technologies Private Ltd.

Koramangala, Bengaluru

Karnataka-560029

http://indiepress.in/

Edited by Ridham Bassi

Typeset by MAP Systems, Bengaluru

Book Cover designed by Nikhil Kamath

Publishing Consultant: Sujhini

Contents

Chapter 1

Introduction

The Vital Role of Nutrition in Health

"The Vital Role of Nutrition in Health" underscores the foundational significance of nutrition in maintaining overall well-being. Nutrition is not merely about satisfying hunger; it is the dynamic process by which the body acquires, processes, and utilizes nutrients to support essential physiological functions.

Cellular Function: Nutrition provides the necessary elements for cellular processes, including energy production, repair, and growth. This is fundamental to maintaining the body's structure and function at the cellular level.

Homeostasis: Proper nutrition is crucial for achieving and maintaining homeostasis – the internal balance necessary for optimal bodily function. It regulates temperature, pH levels, and fluid balance, creating an environment where cells can thrive.

Energy Production: Carbohydrates, fats, and proteins, the macronutrients, are converted into energy through complex biochemical processes. This energy fuels essential bodily functions, from basic metabolic processes to sustaining vital organs.

Cellular Repair and Growth: Proteins, composed of essential amino acids, play a key role in cellular repair, growth, and maintenance. Adequate nutrition ensures the body has the building blocks required for these processes.

Immune System Support: Certain nutrients, such as vitamins and minerals, contribute to the proper functioning of the immune system. A well-nourished body is better equipped to defend itself against infections and diseases.

Cognitive Function: The brain, a metabolically active organ, relies on a steady supply of nutrients for optimal function. Nutrients like omega-3 fatty acids, vitamins B6 and B12, and antioxidants support cognitive function, memory, and emotional well-being.

Preventing Chronic Diseases: Nutrition plays a pivotal role in preventing and managing chronic diseases such as cardiovascular conditions, diabetes, and certain cancers. A balanced and nutrient-rich diet, coupled with a healthy lifestyle, can significantly reduce the risk of these ailments.

Understanding the vital role of nutrition empowers individuals to make informed choices, adopting a proactive approach to well-being. It emphasizes the profound impact that dietary choices have on health, encouraging a holistic perspective that goes beyond mere sustenance.

Evolution of Dietary Science

"The Evolution of Nutrition Science" traces the remarkable journey of nutrition science from its early origins to its current status as a multidisciplinary field. Over the years, the understanding of nutrition has undergone significant transformations, shaped by scientific advancements, societal changes, and a growing awareness of the intricate relationship between diet and health.

Early Observations: The roots of nutrition science can be traced back to ancient civilizations, where early thinkers recognized the connection between certain foods and health. Observations were often based on trial and error and cultural practices.

Discovery of Essential Nutrients: The late 19th and early 20th centuries marked a crucial period when scientists identified essential nutrients like vitamins and minerals. Pioneering figures such as Casimir Funk (who coined the term "vitamin") and Frederick Hopkins laid the groundwork for understanding the role of specific compounds in health.

Deficiency Diseases: The discovery of deficiency diseases, such as scurvy, beriberi, and rickets, provided critical insights into the nutritional requirements of the human body. This period saw the development of nutritional guidelines to address these deficiencies.

World War II and Nutrition: The impact of malnutrition during World War II sparked a renewed interest in nutrition science. Studies on the effects of wartime rationing and the importance of proper nutrition for physical and mental performance contributed to the field's growth.

Emergence of Dietary Guidelines: In the latter half of the 20th century, governments and health organizations began issuing dietary guidelines. These guidelines aimed to educate the public on maintaining health through balanced nutrition and avoiding excesses that could lead to chronic diseases.

Nutrigenomics and Personalized Nutrition: Recent decades have witnessed the rise of nutrigenomics, exploring the interplay between genetics and nutrition. This has paved the way for personalized nutrition, recognizing that individual responses to diet can vary based on genetic factors.

Technological Advances: Advances in technology, including bioinformatics and imaging techniques, have allowed for more sophisticated studies on the effects of nutrients at the molecular and cellular levels. This has expanded our understanding of how nutrition influences health at a granular level.

Holistic Approach: Contemporary nutrition science embraces a holistic approach, acknowledging the interconnectedness of diet, lifestyle, and overall well-being. Researchers now explore the impact of nutrition not only on physical health but also on mental health, chronic diseases, and longevity.

The evolution of nutrition science reflects a continual quest for deeper insights into the complex relationship between what we eat and how it influences our health. From early observations to cutting-edge research, this evolution underscores the dynamic nature of a field that plays a pivotal role in enhancing human health and longevity.

Purpose and Scope of the Book

This books aim to educate readers about the fundamental principles of nutrition, including the roles of various nutrients, dietary guidelines, and the impact of food on overall health. They provide valuable information about the body's nutritional needs and how different foods contribute to well-being.

Chapter 2

Foundations of Nutrition

Macronutrients and Micronutrients

Macronutrients are the essential nutrients that the human body needs in relatively large quantities to function optimally. There are three primary macronutrients: carbohydrates, proteins, and fats.

1. Carbohydrates:

Role: Carbohydrates are the body's main source of energy. They provide fuel for physical activities and support various bodily functions.

Examples:

Simple Carbohydrates: Found in sugars, fruits, and some vegetables.

Complex Carbohydrates: Found in grains, legumes, and starchy vegetables like potatoes.

Impact on Daily Life: Carbohydrates are crucial for sustaining energy levels. They fuel the brain, muscles, and other organs. Including a mix of complex and simple carbohydrates in meals helps maintain stable blood sugar levels, preventing energy crashes.

2. Proteins:

Role: Proteins are essential for the growth, repair, and maintenance of tissues. They also play a role in enzyme and hormone production.

Examples:

Animal Sources: Meat, poultry, fish, eggs, dairy products.

Plant Sources: Legumes (beans, lentils), tofu, nuts, seeds.

Impact on Daily Life: Proteins are vital for muscle development, immune function, and overall tissue health. Including sufficient protein in the diet supports muscle repair after exercise, helps with weight management by promoting satiety, and contributes to the body's structural integrity.

3. Fats:

Role: Fats are a concentrated source of energy. They are essential for cell structure, hormone production, and the absorption of fat-soluble vitamins (A, D, E, K).

Examples:

Healthy Fats: Avocado, olive oil, nuts, seeds, fatty fish.

Unhealthy Fats: Trans fats and saturated fats are found in processed foods and some animal products.

Impact on Daily Life: Healthy fats are crucial for overall health. They contribute to heart health, support brain function, and help in the absorption of vital nutrients. However, excessive intake of unhealthy fats can contribute to weight gain and increase the risk of cardiovascular diseases.

Impact of Macronutrients in Daily Life:

Energy Levels: Adequate macronutrient intake ensures sustained energy throughout the day. Carbohydrates provide quick energy, proteins support endurance, and fats are long-lasting energy sources.

Weight Management: Balancing macronutrients helps regulate appetite and supports healthy weight management. Proteins and fats contribute to feelings of fullness, reducing the likelihood of overeating.

Muscle Health: Protein is essential for muscle repair and growth, making it crucial for individuals engaged in physical activities or those aiming to build muscle mass.

Overall Well-being: A balanced intake of macronutrients is vital for maintaining overall health. It supports immune function, hormone regulation, and the prevention of nutritional deficiencies.

In conclusion, understanding and consciously incorporating a balanced mix of carbohydrates, proteins, and fats into daily meals contribute significantly to overall health, energy levels, and well-being. It's essential to tailor macronutrient intake based on individual needs, activity levels, and health goals.

Understanding Calories

What is a Calorie?

A calorie is a unit of measurement for energy. In the context of nutrition, the term "calorie" is often used to quantify the amount of energy provided by food and beverages. It represents the amount of heat energy needed to raise the temperature of one gram of water by one degree Celsius. In nutritional terms, calories are used to express the energy content of the food we consume.

How is it Calculated?

The calorie content of food is determined through a process called calorimetry. In a bomb calorimeter, a food sample is burned, and the heat produced is measured. This measurement is then converted into units of energy, providing an estimate of the food's caloric content. However, for practical purposes in nutrition, the calorie content of food is often calculated using the Atwater system, which assigns specific values to each gram of protein, carbohydrates, and fats.

Proteins: 1 gram = 4 calories

Carbohydrates: 1 gram = 4 calories

Fats: 1 gram = 9 calories

Alcohol: 1 gram = 7 calories

These values are averages and provide a reasonable estimate of the energy content of different macronutrients.

From where do we get Calories?

Calories come from the macronutrients present in the foods and beverages we consume:

Carbohydrates: Found in grains, fruits, vegetables, legumes, and sugars.

Proteins: Found in meat, poultry, fish, dairy products, legumes, nuts, and seeds.

Fats: Found in oils, butter, avocados, nuts, seeds, and fatty fish.

Alcohol: Found in alcoholic beverages.

Each of these macronutrients provides a specific amount of calories per gram, as mentioned earlier.

Impact of Calories in Daily Lives:

Energy Balance: Calories are essential for providing the energy needed to carry out daily activities, from basic bodily functions like breathing and maintaining body temperature to more active pursuits like exercise.

Weight Management: The balance between the number of calories consumed and the number of calories expended influences body weight. Consuming more calories than the body needs leads to weight gain, while a calorie deficit results in weight loss.

Nutrient Intake: Monitoring calorie intake helps ensure that the body receives an appropriate amount of essential nutrients. A balanced diet with the right proportion of macronutrients supports overall health and well-being.

Physical Performance: Athletes and individuals engaged in physical activities need to manage their calorie intake to meet energy demands and support optimal performance and recovery.

Metabolic Health: The type of calories consumed (nutrient-dense vs. empty calories) can impact metabolic health. Poor dietary choices may contribute to conditions like obesity and related metabolic disorders.

In summary, calories are a fundamental aspect of nutrition, representing the energy derived from the foods we eat. Understanding and managing calorie intake are crucial for maintaining a healthy weight, supporting physical activity, and promoting overall well-being.

The Importance of Hydration

1. Essential for Survival:

Water is fundamental for life, and adequate hydration is essential for the survival of all living organisms, including humans. Dehydration, or insufficient water intake, can lead to serious health issues and, in extreme cases, can be life-threatening.

2. Supports Bodily Functions:

Water plays a crucial role in various physiological functions, including digestion, absorption of nutrients, and the transportation of oxygen and other essential substances throughout the body. It is a key component of bodily fluids, including blood and lymph.

3. Temperature Regulation:

Sweating is the body's natural mechanism for cooling down. Adequate hydration helps regulate body temperature by facilitating the evaporation of sweat, preventing overheating during physical activity or exposure to high temperatures.

4. Cognitive Function:

Dehydration can impair cognitive function, affecting concentration, alertness, and short-term memory. Staying hydrated supports optimal brain function, improving mental clarity and overall cognitive performance.

5. Joint and Tissue Lubrication:

Water serves as a lubricant for joints and tissues, facilitating smooth movement and reducing friction. Proper hydration is crucial for joint health and can help prevent conditions like arthritis and muscle cramps.

6. Skin Health:

Hydration is essential for maintaining skin elasticity and preventing dryness. Well-hydrated skin looks healthier, feels smoother, and is more resistant to the effects of aging.

7. Waste Elimination:

Water is a key component in the body's waste elimination process. It helps flush out toxins and waste products through urine, supporting the health of the kidneys and the urinary system.

8. Energy Production:

Hydration is necessary for efficient energy production within cells. Water is involved in various metabolic processes, including the breakdown of nutrients to produce energy. Dehydration can lead to feelings of fatigue and decreased physical performance.

9. Exercise Performance:

Athletes and individuals engaged in physical activity require adequate hydration to maintain endurance, strength, and overall performance. Dehydration during exercise can lead to muscle cramps, heat-related illnesses, and a decrease in exercise capacity.

10. Immune System Support:

Hydration plays a role in supporting the immune system. Well-hydrated individuals are better equipped to fend off infections and recover more efficiently from illnesses.

11. Weight Management:

Drinking water before meals can contribute to a feeling of fullness, potentially reducing overall calorie intake and supporting weight management efforts.

12. Electrolyte Balance:

Electrolytes, such as sodium, potassium, and chloride, are essential for various physiological processes. Hydration helps maintain the balance of electrolytes in the body, which is crucial for nerve function, muscle contractions, and fluid balance.

Tips for Hydration:

- Drink an adequate amount of water throughout the day, adjusting intake based on factors like age, activity level, and climate.

- Monitor urine color; pale yellow indicates proper hydration.

- Consume hydrating foods, such as fruits and vegetables, with high water content.

- Be mindful of hydration needs during physical activity, illness, or exposure to hot weather.

In conclusion, maintaining proper hydration is essential for overall health and well-being, impacting numerous bodily functions and supporting optimal performance in various aspects of life. Regular and sufficient water intake is a simple yet crucial aspect of a healthy lifestyle.

Understanding BMR

Basal Metabolic Rate (BMR) is a fundamental concept in the realm of human metabolism, playing a crucial role in determining how many calories our bodies burn at rest. This metric holds significant importance in various fields, including fitness, nutrition, and weight management. In this article, we will delve into the intricacies of BMR, its significance, the factors influencing it, and how it can be utilized to achieve health and fitness goals.

What is Basal Metabolic Rate (BMR)?

BMR represents the minimum amount of energy or calories that the body requires at rest to maintain basic physiological functions such as breathing, circulation, and cell production. It is often expressed as calories per day and is influenced by factors like age, gender, body composition, and genetics. Understanding BMR is pivotal for comprehending the baseline energy needs of an individual.

Factors Influencing BMR:

Age: BMR tends to decrease with age, primarily due to a decline in muscle mass and a decrease in metabolic activity.

Gender: Men generally have a higher BMR than women, primarily because men tend to have more muscle mass, which requires more energy at rest.

Body Composition: Muscle tissue is more metabolically active than fat tissue. Therefore, individuals with higher muscle mass typically have a higher BMR.

Genetics: Genetic factors can influence metabolic rate, affecting how efficiently the body burns calories.

Hormones: Thyroid hormones, especially thyroxine (T4) and triiodothyronine (T3), play a crucial role in regulating BMR.

Calculating BMR:

Several formulas are used to estimate BMR. The Harris-Benedict equation is one of the most commonly employed methods, taking into account factors like age, gender, weight, and height. An example for men is:

BMR=88.362+(13.397×weight in kg)+(4.799×height in cm)-(5.677×age in years)

For women, the equation is slightly different:

BMR=447.593+(9.247×weight in kg)+(3.098×height in cm)-(4.330×age in years)*BMR*=447.593+(9.247×weight in kg)+(3.098×height in cm)-(4.330×age in years)

Significance of BMR in Weight Management:

Understanding one's BMR is essential for creating effective weight management strategies. If calorie intake exceeds BMR, weight gain is likely, while a calorie deficit leads to weight loss. By incorporating BMR into dietary planning, individuals can tailor their calorie intake to achieve specific health and fitness goals.

Practical Applications of BMR:

Weight Loss: Creating a calorie deficit by consuming fewer calories than the BMR helps shed excess body weight.

Weight Maintenance: Adjusting calorie intake to match BMR supports maintaining a stable weight.

Muscle Building: Individuals looking to build muscle can utilize BMR to determine their calorie needs, ensuring sufficient energy for muscle growth.

Basal Metabolic Rate is a key determinant in the complex web of human metabolism. Recognizing its role in energy balance empowers individuals to make informed decisions about their nutrition and fitness goals. Whether aiming for weight loss, maintenance, or muscle gain, incorporating BMR into lifestyle choices can pave the way for a healthier and more balanced life.

Chapter 3

Building a Balanced Plate

Building a balanced plate in nutrition refers to creating a meal that provides a mix of essential nutrients in appropriate proportions to support overall health and well-being. A balanced plate typically includes a combination of macronutrients (carbohydrates, proteins, and fats) along with micronutrients (vitamins and minerals) to ensure that the body receives the necessary nutrients for optimal functioning.

Here are some general guidelines for building a balanced plate:

1. Incorporate a Variety of Foods:

Include a variety of food groups to ensure a diverse range of nutrients. This may include fruits, vegetables, whole grains, lean proteins, and healthy fats.

2. Balanced Macronutrients:

Include a source of carbohydrates, proteins, and fats in each meal.

Carbohydrates: Whole grains, fruits, and vegetables.

Proteins: lean meats, poultry, fish, tofu, legumes, and dairy products.

Fats: Healthy fats from sources like avocados, nuts, seeds, and olive oil.

3. Watch Portion Sizes:

Pay attention to portion sizes to avoid overeating. Balancing the amounts of different food groups can help control calorie intake and maintain a healthy weight.

4. Colorful Plate:

Aim for a colorful plate by including a variety of fruits and vegetables. Different colors often indicate a variety of nutrients, so a colorful plate is a good indicator of nutritional diversity.

5. Whole Foods vs. Processed Foods:

Prioritize whole, minimally processed foods over highly processed ones. Whole foods tend to be more nutrient-dense and provide a broader range of essential nutrients.

6. Hydration:

Don't forget about hydration. Water is an essential component of a balanced diet. Include water or other healthy beverages to stay well-hydrated.

7. Mindful Eating:

Practice mindful eating by paying attention to hunger and fullness cues. This helps prevent overeating and encourages a healthier relationship with food.

8. Consider Individual Needs:

Individual nutritional needs vary based on factors such as age, sex, activity level, and health conditions. Adjust the balance of nutrients based on individual requirements and goals.

Building a balanced plate is a practical way to ensure that your meals provide the necessary nutrients for energy, growth, and overall well-being. By including a variety of nutrient-dense foods in appropriate portions, you can support optimal health and meet your nutritional needs. Keep in mind that these are general guidelines, and consulting with a registered dietitian or healthcare professional can provide personalized advice based on individual requirements and health goals.

The Mediterranean Diet

The Mediterranean diet is a dietary pattern inspired by the traditional eating habits of populations in countries bordering the Mediterranean Sea, such as Greece, Italy, and Spain. It has gained recognition for its potential health benefits and is often recommended by health professionals. The Mediterranean diet is characterized by several key features:

1. Emphasis on Plant-Based Foods:

The majority of the diet comes from plant-based sources, including fruits, vegetables, whole grains, legumes, nuts, and seeds.

2. Olive Oil as the Primary Fat:

Olive oil is the main source of fat in the Mediterranean diet. It is rich in monounsaturated fats, which are considered heart-healthy.

3. Moderate Consumption of Fish and Poultry:

Fish and poultry are recommended over red meat. Fatty fish, such as salmon and mackerel, are particularly encouraged due to their omega-3 fatty acids.

4. Limited Red Meat and Dairy:

Red meat and dairy products are consumed in moderation. The focus is on lean proteins and low-fat dairy options when included.

5. Herbs and Spices for Flavor:

Herbs and spices are used to add flavor to dishes instead of relying heavily on salt. This contributes to the diet's overall healthfulness.

6. Regular Intake of Fruits and Nuts:

Fruits and nuts are important components of the Mediterranean diet, providing essential vitamins, minerals, and healthy fats.

7. Moderate Wine Consumption:

Moderate consumption of red wine is often associated with the Mediterranean diet. This is typically one glass per day for women and up to two glasses per day for men, consumed with meals.

8. Regular Physical Activity:

Physical activity is considered an integral part of the Mediterranean lifestyle. Regular exercise complements the dietary pattern for overall health.

Nutritional Benefits of the Mediterranean Diet:

Heart Health:

The Mediterranean diet is associated with a reduced risk of heart disease. The emphasis on olive oil, fish, and a variety of plant-based foods contributes to cardiovascular health.

Weight Management:

The diet's focus on whole, nutrient-dense foods and portion control supports healthy weight management.

Cancer Prevention:

Some studies suggest that the Mediterranean diet may be associated with a lower risk of certain cancers, particularly colorectal cancer.

Diabetes Management:

The diet's emphasis on whole grains, fruits, and vegetables may help manage blood sugar levels and reduce the risk of type 2 diabetes.

Brain Health:

The inclusion of omega-3 fatty acids from fish, as well as antioxidants from fruits and vegetables, is thought to support brain health and reduce the risk of cognitive decline.

Longevity:

Populations following a Mediterranean diet have been associated with increased longevity and a lower risk of age-related diseases.

It's important to note that the Mediterranean diet is a general dietary pattern, and individual variations exist. Moreover, lifestyle factors such as regular physical activity and social interactions contribute to the overall health benefits associated with this eating pattern. Before making significant changes to your diet, it's advisable to consult with a healthcare professional or a registered dietitian to ensure that it aligns with your individual health needs and goals.

Plant-Based vs. Animal-Based Diets

The realm of nutrition is rife with discussions about the merits of plant-based diets versus their animal-based counterparts. As individuals become more conscious of their health, environmental impact, and ethical considerations, the debate between these two dietary approaches has gained prominence. In this article, we'll delve into the characteristics, benefits, and potential drawbacks of plant-based and animal-based diets to provide a comprehensive overview.

Plant-Based Diets:

Plant-based diets predominantly focus on foods derived from plants, such as fruits, vegetables, whole grains, nuts, seeds, and legumes. The emphasis is on consuming nutrient-dense, fiber-rich foods while minimizing or eliminating animal products.

Benefits of Plant-Based Diets:

Nutrient Density: Plant-based diets are rich in vitamins, minerals, and antioxidants, contributing to overall health and well-being.

Heart Health: Studies suggest that plant-based diets may lower the risk of heart disease, reduce cholesterol levels, and improve blood pressure.

Weight Management: The high fiber content of plant-based foods can promote satiety and support weight management by reducing overall calorie intake.

Environmental Impact: Plant-based diets are often touted for their lower environmental footprint, as plant agriculture generally requires fewer resources compared to animal agriculture.

Ethical Considerations: Many individuals adopt plant-based diets for ethical reasons, such as concerns about animal welfare and the environmental impact of livestock farming.

Drawbacks of Plant-Based Diets:

Nutrient Deficiencies: Without proper planning, plant-based diets may lack certain nutrients, such as vitamin B12, iron, zinc, and omega-3 fatty acids, which are more abundantly found in animal products.

Protein Sources: While plant-based sources of protein exist, individuals must be mindful to consume a variety of protein-rich foods to meet their protein needs.

Animal-Based Diets:

Animal-based diets, on the other hand, include a variety of animal products such as meat, poultry, fish, eggs, and dairy. These diets may vary in their composition, with some emphasizing lean proteins and others incorporating higher levels of saturated fats.

Benefits of Animal-Based Diets:

Complete Proteins: Animal products provide complete proteins, containing all essential amino acids necessary for muscle growth and repair.

Nutrient Bioavailability: Animal-based sources are rich in heme iron, vitamin B12, and other nutrients that are more readily absorbed by the body compared to some plant-based sources.

Muscle Mass and Strength: The amino acid profile of animal proteins is often associated with better support for muscle mass and strength.

Convenience: Animal products are often more convenient for individuals who have busy lifestyles, as they provide quick and concentrated sources of nutrition.

Drawbacks of Animal-Based Diets:

Heart Health Concerns: Some animal-based diets, particularly those high in saturated fats, may be associated with an increased risk of heart disease.

Environmental Impact: Livestock farming contributes significantly to environmental issues such as deforestation, greenhouse gas emissions, and water pollution.

Ethical Concerns: Animal welfare issues, including factory farming practices, can raise ethical concerns for individuals opting for a more compassionate approach to food choices.

The debate between plant-based and animal-based diets is nuanced and multifaceted. Ultimately, the choice between these dietary approaches should consider individual health goals, ethical considerations, and environmental impact. Many experts suggest that a well-balanced diet, regardless of its primary source, can meet nutritional needs. Consulting with a healthcare professional or registered dietitian is advisable for personalized dietary guidance based on individual health factors and lifestyle choices.

Plant-Based vs. Animal-Based Diets: Which is better?

The question of whether a plant-based or animal-based diet is "better" is complex and depends on various factors, including individual health goals, ethical considerations, environmental concerns, and personal preferences. Both types of diets have their advantages and potential drawbacks, and what works best for one person may not be suitable for another. Let's explore the pros and cons of each to provide a more nuanced understanding:

Plant-Based Diet:

Pros:

Rich in Nutrients: Plant-based diets are often rich in vitamins, minerals, antioxidants, and fiber, which contribute to overall health and well-being.

Heart Health: Studies suggest that plant-based diets may be associated with a reduced risk of heart disease due to lower saturated fat intake and higher consumption of heart-healthy foods like fruits, vegetables, and whole grains.

Environmental Impact: Plant-based diets generally have a lower environmental footprint, as they require fewer resources and produce fewer greenhouse gas emissions compared to animal agriculture.

Ethical Considerations: Many individuals adopt plant-based diets for ethical reasons, such as concerns about animal welfare and the environmental impact of livestock farming.

Cons:

Nutrient Deficiencies: Without careful planning, plant-based diets may lack certain nutrients commonly found in animal products, such as vitamin B12, iron, zinc, and omega-3 fatty acids.

Protein Sources: While plant-based protein sources exist, individuals need to ensure they consume a variety of protein-rich foods to meet their protein needs.

Animal-Based Diet:

Pros:

Complete Proteins: Animal products provide complete proteins containing all essential amino acids necessary for muscle growth and repair.

Nutrient Bioavailability: Nutrients from animal products, such as heme iron and vitamin B12, are often more readily absorbed by the body compared to some plant-based sources.

Muscle Mass and Strength: The amino acid profile of animal proteins is associated with better support for muscle mass and strength.

Cons:

Heart Health Concerns: Diets high in saturated fats from animal products may be associated with an increased risk of heart disease.

Environmental Impact: Livestock farming contributes significantly to environmental issues such as deforestation, greenhouse gas emissions, and water pollution.

Ethical Concerns: Some individuals choose to avoid animal products due to concerns about factory farming practices and animal welfare.

There is no one-size-fits-all answer to the question of whether a plant-based or an animal-based diet is better. It's crucial to consider individual health needs, ethical beliefs, and environmental considerations. Many experts advocate for a balanced approach, incorporating a variety of foods to ensure a diverse nutrient intake. Consulting with a healthcare professional or registered dietitian can provide personalized guidance based on individual factors and goals. Ultimately, the "better" diet is the one that aligns with an individual's values, promotes overall well-being, and is sustainable in the long term.

Portion Control and Mindful Eating

Portion Control:

Portion control refers to managing the quantity of food served and consumed in a single meal or snack. It involves being mindful of the amount of food on the plate and avoiding overeating. Portion control is essential for maintaining a healthy weight, preventing overconsumption of calories, and ensuring a balanced intake of nutrients.

Key Aspects of Portion Control Include:

Understanding Serving Sizes: Recognizing and understanding recommended serving sizes for different food groups to avoid excessive calorie intake.

Using Visual Cues: Using visual cues, such as portion control tools or comparing food portions to familiar objects (e.g., a deck of cards for meat), to estimate appropriate serving sizes.

Avoiding Super-sized Portions: Being conscious of portion sizes when dining out, as restaurant portions are often larger than necessary for a single meal.

Listening to Hunger and Fullness Cues: Paying attention to feelings of hunger and fullness and stopping eating when satisfied, rather than when the plate is empty.

Choosing Nutrient-Dense Foods: Opting for nutrient-dense foods in appropriate portions to meet nutritional needs without excessive calories.

Mindful Eating:

Mindful eating involves being fully present and attentive during meals, paying attention to the sensory experience of eating, and fostering a non-judgmental awareness of one's thoughts and feelings related to food. It goes beyond portion control and extends to the overall eating experience, promoting a healthier relationship with food.

Key Aspects of Mindful Eating Include:

Eating with Awareness: Being present in the moment while eating, savoring flavors, textures, and aromas, and appreciating the overall dining experience.

Recognizing Hunger and Fullness: Listening to the body's hunger and fullness cues and eating in response to physiological hunger rather than emotional triggers.

Avoiding Distractions: Minimizing distractions such as television, phones, or computers during meals to focus on the act of eating and the enjoyment of food.

Chewing Thoroughly: Taking the time to chew food thoroughly, which aids in digestion and allows the body to recognize fullness.

Non-Judgmental Awareness: Approaching food choices without judgment or guilt, recognizing that food is neither "good" nor "bad," but rather a source of nourishment.

Learning to Cope with Emotions: Developing awareness of emotional eating patterns and finding alternative ways to cope with stress, boredom, or other emotions.

Both portion control and mindful eating are complementary approaches that contribute to a healthy and balanced relationship with food. Combining these practices can support overall well-being, weight management, and the enjoyment of meals.

Chapter 4

Nutrition Across the Lifespan

Nutrition Across the Lifespan: A Vital Pillar for Health and Well-Being

Nutrition is a fundamental aspect of human development and plays a pivotal role in ensuring optimal health across the lifespan. From the earliest stages of life to the golden years of seniority, the quality of nutrition profoundly influences growth, cognitive development, and overall well-being.

In the realm of prenatal nutrition, the significance of a mother's diet extends beyond her own health to that of the growing fetus. Adequate intake of essential nutrients like folic acid, iron, and calcium during pregnancy is crucial for preventing birth defects, supporting fetal growth, and laying the foundation for a healthy life.

As individuals transition into childhood, nutrition remains a key determinant of physical and cognitive development. The early years are characterized by rapid growth, and a well-balanced diet rich in calcium, protein, iron, and fiber is essential for the formation of healthy bones, organs, and neural pathways. Establishing healthy eating habits during childhood sets the stage for a lifetime of well-being.

The adolescent years bring about unique nutritional needs due to growth spurts and hormonal changes. Adequate intake of calcium and vitamin D supports bone health during this critical phase, while sufficient protein ensures proper muscle development. Nutrient-dense foods become paramount, laying the groundwork for a healthy transition into adulthood.

In adulthood, nutrition continues to play a central role in sustaining overall health and preventing chronic diseases. A balanced diet that includes a variety of fruits, vegetables, whole grains, and lean proteins supports energy levels, weight management, and the body's ability to ward off illnesses. Proper nutrition is not only a factor in physical health but also has implications for mental well-being and cognitive function.

As individuals reach their senior years, nutritional needs evolve, and a focus on specific nutrients becomes essential. Adequate intake of calcium and vitamin D remains vital for maintaining bone health, while attention to protein helps prevent the loss of muscle mass associated with aging. Fiber-rich foods support digestive health, and sufficient hydration becomes increasingly important.

Throughout this journey, the role of nutrition is not only about providing sustenance but also about preventing nutritional deficiencies and promoting overall health. The interplay between diet and health is a dynamic and intricate relationship that underscores the importance of mindful eating habits and nutrition education at every life stage.

In conclusion, the significance of nutrition across the lifespan cannot be overstated. It is the cornerstone of a healthy, vibrant life, impacting growth, development, and the prevention of diseases. Embracing a balanced and nutrient-dense diet from the earliest stages of life ensures not only physical well-being but also sets the stage for a fulfilling and healthy journey through the various chapters of life.

Prenatal Nutrition

Key Nutrients:

1. Folic Acid:

- Importance: crucial for neural tube development in the fetus, preventing birth defects.
- Food Sources: leafy greens, fortified cereals, beans.

2. Iron:

- Importance: vital for preventing maternal anemia and supporting fetal growth.
- Food Sources: red meat, poultry, fish, beans, fortified cereals.

3. Calcium:

- Importance: essential for bone development in the fetus.
- Food Sources: dairy products, leafy greens, fortified plant-based milk.

4. Omega-3 Fatty Acids:

- Importance: support brain and vision development in the fetus.
- Food Sources: fatty fish (salmon, trout), chia seeds, walnuts.

Recommendations:

- Adequate intake of prenatal vitamins.
- A well-balanced diet with a focus on fruits, vegetables, whole grains, and lean proteins.
- Limited caffeine intake.
- Avoidance of certain foods, such as raw seafood and unpasteurized dairy.
- Childhood Nutrition:

Key Nutrients:

1. Calcium and Vitamin D:

- Importance: crucial for bone development in growing children.
- Food Sources: dairy products, fortified cereals, fatty fish.

2. Protein:

- Importance: essential for growth and development.
- Food Sources: lean meat, poultry, dairy, beans, nuts.

3. Iron:

- Importance: important for cognitive development and preventing anemia.
- Food Sources: red meat, poultry, beans, fortified cereals.

4. Fiber:

- Importance: supports digestive health and helps prevent constipation.
- Food Sources: fruits, vegetables, whole grains, legumes.

Recommendations:

- Encouragement of a balanced diet including a variety of fruits, vegetables, whole grains, and lean proteins.
- Limiting added sugars and processed foods.
- Adequate hydration to support growth and development.
- Nutrition for Adolescents:

Key Nutrients:

1. Calcium and Vitamin D:

- Importance: important for bone health during growth spurts.
- Food Sources: dairy products, fortified plant-based milk, leafy greens.

2. Protein:

- Importance: essential for growth and muscle development.
- Food Sources: lean meat, poultry, fish, dairy, plant-based protein sources.

3. Iron:

- Importance: particularly important for menstruating females.
- Food Sources: red meat, poultry, beans, fortified cereals.

4. Folate and B Vitamins:

- Importance: support energy levels and cognitive function.
- Food Sources: whole grains, leafy greens, fortified cereals, nuts.

Recommendations:

- Emphasis on nutrient-dense foods to support growth and development.
- Education on balanced eating habits and the importance of hydration.
- Monitoring of iron levels, especially for females.
- Adult Nutrition:

Key Nutrients:

1. Protein:

- Importance: important for maintaining muscle mass and overall health.
- Food Sources: lean meat, poultry, fish, dairy, plant-based protein sources.

2. Calcium and Vitamin D:

- Importance: essential for bone health and maintenance.
- Food Sources: dairy products, fortified plant-based milk, leafy greens.

3. Fiber:

- Importance: supports digestive health, weight management, and heart health.
- Food Sources: fruits, vegetables, whole grains, legumes.

4. Omega-3 Fatty Acids:

- Importance: support heart health and cognitive function.
- Food Sources: fatty fish, flaxseeds, chia seeds, walnuts.

Recommendations:

- Balanced diet with a variety of nutrients from different food groups.

- Portion control and moderation to prevent overconsumption.
- Adequate hydration and mindful eating.
- Senior Nutrition:

Key Nutrients:

1. Calcium and Vitamin D:

- Importance: vital for maintaining bone health and preventing fractures.
- Food Sources: dairy products, fortified plant-based milk, leafy greens.

2. Protein:

- Importance: important for maintaining muscle mass and preventing sarcopenia.
- Food Sources: lean meat, poultry, fish, dairy, plant-based protein sources.

3. Fiber:

- Importance: supports digestive health and prevents constipation.
- Food Sources: fruits, vegetables, whole grains, legumes.

4. Vitamin B12:

- Importance: essential for nerve function.
- Food Sources: meat, fish, dairy, fortified cereals.

Recommendations:

- Focus on nutrient-dense foods due to potential decreased calorie needs.
- Regular monitoring of vitamin and mineral levels.
- Adequate hydration and consideration of dietary restrictions or health conditions.

Understanding these nutritional needs at different life stages is crucial for promoting health, preventing nutritional deficiencies, and ensuring overall well-being. Individual variations and health conditions may require personalized nutrition plans, and consulting with healthcare professionals is advisable for tailored guidance.

Chapter 5

Functional Foods and Superfoods

Functional foods and superfoods are terms often used to describe foods that offer additional health benefits beyond their basic nutritional value. These foods are believed to have properties that contribute to overall well-being and may help prevent or manage certain health conditions.

Functional Foods:

Definition:

Functional foods are those that provide health benefits beyond basic nutrition due to the specific bioactive compounds they contain.

Examples:

Probiotics: Yogurt, kefir, and fermented foods contain live beneficial bacteria that support gut health.

Omega-3 Fatty Acid-Rich Foods: Fatty fish (salmon, mackerel), flaxseeds, and walnuts contribute to heart health and may have anti-inflammatory effects.

Fortified Foods: These foods are enriched with additional nutrients, such as calcium-fortified orange juice or vitamin D-fortified milk.

Health Benefits:

Digestive Health: Probiotics in functional foods can promote a healthy balance of gut bacteria.

Heart Health: Omega-3 fatty acids may reduce the risk of cardiovascular diseases.

Bone Health: Calcium-fortified foods contribute to bone strength.

Superfoods:

Superfoods refer to nutrient-dense foods that are rich in vitamins, minerals, and antioxidants.

Examples:

Berries: Blueberries, strawberries, and acai berries are high in antioxidants.

Leafy Greens: Kale, spinach, and Swiss chard are rich in vitamins and minerals.

Nuts and Seeds: Almonds, chia seeds, and flax seeds provide healthy fats and essential nutrients.

Health Benefits:

Antioxidant Protection: Superfoods are often rich in antioxidants that help combat oxidative stress and inflammation.

Nutrient Density: They provide a high concentration of essential nutrients while relatively low in calories.

Heart Health: Certain superfoods, like nuts and berries, may contribute to cardiovascular health.

Important Considerations:

While both functional foods and superfoods offer health benefits, it's essential to maintain a balanced diet that includes a variety of nutrient-rich foods. The terms "functional" and "superfood" are not regulated, and marketing hype can sometimes exaggerate their benefits. A diverse and well-rounded diet, combined with a healthy lifestyle, is key to overall health.

Incorporating a mix of functional foods and superfoods into a balanced diet can contribute to better health. However, it's crucial to consult with healthcare professionals or registered dietitians for personalized advice, especially if addressing specific health concerns or conditions.

Exploring the Power of Superfoods

The Power of Functional Foods: Unlocking Health Benefits Beyond Nutrition

Functional Foods, often heralded as nutritional powerhouses, are redefining our approach to diet and well-being. These foods go beyond the basic role of providing sustenance; they are enriched with bioactive compounds that offer a spectrum of health benefits. By incorporating functional foods into our diets, we tap into a potent resource that supports and enhances various aspects of our health.

1. Gut Health and Probiotics:

Functional foods rich in probiotics, such as yogurt, kefir, and fermented foods, contribute to a thriving ecosystem of beneficial bacteria in the gut. This balance, known as the microbiome, plays a crucial role in digestion, nutrient absorption, and even immune function. The power of these foods lies in their ability to promote a healthy gut, potentially reducing the risk of gastrointestinal issues and bolstering overall well-being.

2. Omega-3 Fatty Acids for Heart Health:

Fatty fish like salmon, flaxseeds, and walnuts are rich in omega-3 fatty acids—a nutritional treasure for cardiovascular health. These functional foods exhibit anti-inflammatory properties, help regulate cholesterol levels, and support optimal heart function. By incorporating them into our diets, we harness the power to reduce the risk of heart disease and promote a healthier cardiovascular system.

3. Antioxidant-Rich Superfoods:

Superfoods, brimming with antioxidants, possess the power to combat oxidative stress and inflammation within the body. Berries, kale, and nuts are among the superfoods celebrated for their nutrient density and disease-fighting capabilities. Antioxidants play a crucial role in neutralizing free radicals, contributing to cellular health, and potentially lowering the risk of chronic conditions.

4. Fortified Foods for Nutrient Boost:

Functional foods such as fortified cereals, dairy products, and plant-based milk alternatives are designed to address specific nutritional needs. These foods are fortified with additional vitamins and minerals, providing a convenient way to bridge nutritional gaps. The power lies in their ability to enhance the nutrient profile of commonly consumed foods, supporting overall health and vitality.

5. Balancing Blood Sugar with Fiber:

Functional foods rich in soluble fiber, such as oats, legumes, and certain fruits, play a crucial role in regulating blood sugar levels. The power of fiber extends beyond digestive health—it helps manage insulin sensitivity, making these foods valuable for individuals with diabetes or those aiming to maintain stable blood sugar levels.

6. Cognitive Support with Brain-Boosting Foods:

Certain functional foods, including fatty fish, nuts, and berries, are recognized for their potential to support cognitive function. Omega-3 fatty acids and antioxidants in these foods contribute to brain health, potentially reducing the risk of age-related cognitive decline. The power here lies in the synergy of nutrients that nourish and protect the brain.

The power of functional foods resides in their ability to provide not just sustenance but an added layer of health benefits. Incorporating these foods into a well-balanced diet offers a proactive approach to health, empowering individuals to optimize their well-being and potentially reduce the risk of various health conditions. However, it's essential to approach dietary choices holistically, considering individual health needs and consulting with healthcare professionals or registered dietitians for personalized guidance.

The Importance of Balance:

While the power of functional foods is undeniable, it is essential to emphasize the importance of a balanced diet. No single food or group of foods can provide all the nutrients the body needs. A well-rounded and diverse diet that includes a variety of functional foods, along with other nutrient-dense options, is key to achieving optimal health.

Integrating Functional Foods into Your Diet

In the quest for optimal health, the spotlight is increasingly turning towards functional foods—a category of edibles that goes beyond basic nutrition, offering a treasure trove of health benefits. Integrating these powerhouse foods into your diet isn't just a culinary trend; it's a strategic move for enhancing overall well-being. Let's delve into the compelling reasons why incorporating functional foods is pivotal for your health journey.

1. Nutrient-Rich Powerhouses:

Functional foods are nutrient-dense and packed with a symphony of vitamins, minerals, and antioxidants. They amplify the nutritional value of your meals, ensuring that every bite contributes substantially to your daily nutrient requirements.

2. Disease Defense and Prevention:

The allure of functional foods lies in their potential to shield against chronic diseases. Imagine your diet as a shield—fortified by functional foods, it becomes a powerful defense mechanism.

Example: Fatty fish, a functional food abundant in omega-3 fatty acids, is renowned for promoting heart health and reducing the risk of cardiovascular diseases.

3. Gut Harmony and Digestive Bliss:

A harmonious gut translates to a healthier you. Functional foods with probiotics and prebiotics foster a thriving gut microbiome, promoting efficient digestion and nutrient absorption.

Example: Incorporating yogurt, a probiotic-rich functional food, can cultivate a diverse and balanced gut flora.

4. Elevated Energy and Cognitive Clarity:

Experience sustained energy levels and heightened cognitive function with the right nutritional choices. Functional foods contribute to mental clarity and focus, empowering you to tackle daily challenges.

Example: Berries, bursting with antioxidants, have been linked to improved cognitive function and memory retention.

5. Guardians of Antioxidant Defense:

Functional foods, often labeled as superfoods, are armed with antioxidants that combat cellular damage. This defense mechanism plays a crucial role in preventing various diseases and supporting overall cellular health.

Example: Kale, a renowned superfood, is a powerhouse of antioxidants, safeguarding your body against oxidative stress.

6. Holistic Wellness Approach:

The integration of functional foods invites a holistic approach to wellness. Rather than targeting specific issues, these foods contribute to overall health, addressing multiple facets of well-being.

Example: Turmeric, known for its anti-inflammatory properties, doesn't just address inflammation but contributes to the overall balance of the body.

7. Versatility Meets Culinary Joy:

Functional foods seamlessly blend into various culinary creations, making healthy eating an enjoyable journey. The versatility of these foods allows you to experiment with flavors and textures, ensuring your meals are both nutritious and delightful.

Example: Quinoa, a functional food rich in protein and fiber, can star in salads, serve as a side dish, or even take center stage in a hearty bowl.

The integration of functional foods into your diet is not just a dietary choice; it's a proactive step towards a healthier, more vibrant you. These foods are not mere ingredients; they are nutritional powerhouses that, when embraced, unlock a spectrum of health benefits. So, embark on this flavorful journey, explore the diverse world of functional foods, and savor the holistic well-being they bring to your plate and your life.

Myth vs. Reality: Superfood Hype

Navigating the Superfood Hype

The term "superfood" has become a nutritional buzzword, enticing health enthusiasts with promises of extraordinary health benefits. However, behind the superfood hype lies a landscape of myths and realities that need careful navigation. Let's dissect the common myths surrounding superfoods and uncover the realities that shape a more balanced understanding of these nutritionally dense edibles.

Myth 1: Superfoods Can Cure Everything

Reality: While superfoods are nutrient powerhouses, the idea that they can single-handedly cure ailments is a myth. The concept of a "magic bullet" in nutrition oversimplifies the complex interplay of factors that contribute to health. Superfoods should be seen as part of a holistic and varied diet that, when combined with a healthy lifestyle, contributes to overall well-being.

Myth 2: Superfoods are Exotic and Expensive

Reality: The image of superfoods as rare, exotic, and costly is a misconception. Many everyday, affordable foods are just as nutrient-rich as those with a superfood label. Local produce, such as spinach, blueberries, and beans, is packed with vitamins and antioxidants. A well-rounded diet that includes a variety of foods is more important than chasing after expensive exotic options.

Myth 3: Superfoods Guarantee Weight Loss

Reality: No single food guarantees weight loss. While some superfoods may aid in weight management due to their nutrient density and fiber content, they are not a magic solution. Weight loss is a complex process involving a combination of factors, including an overall diet, physical activity, and individual metabolism.

Myth 4: Superfoods Alone Make a Healthy Diet

Reality: Incorporating superfoods is beneficial, but a truly healthy diet requires diversity. Relying solely on a handful of superfoods neglects the importance of a broad spectrum of nutrients from different food groups. A balanced diet includes fruits, vegetables, whole grains, lean proteins, and healthy fats.

Myth 5: Superfoods Are Always Better in Supplement Form

Reality: While supplements can be convenient, they may lack the synergistic effects of nutrients found in whole foods. The combination of vitamins, minerals, fiber, and other compounds in whole foods provides a holistic nutritional package that supplements might not replicate.

Myth 6: Superfoods Can Compensate for an Unhealthy Lifestyle

Reality: No amount of superfoods can offset the negative effects of an unhealthy lifestyle. Regular exercise, sufficient sleep, and stress management are integral components of well-being. Relying solely on superfoods while neglecting these lifestyle factors is an incomplete approach to health.

The superfood hype has undoubtedly brought attention to nutrient-rich foods, but it's crucial to separate myth from reality. Superfoods are part of a broader strategy for maintaining good health, and a balanced, varied diet is the key. Rather than fixating on individual foods, adopting a holistic approach to nutrition, combined with a healthy lifestyle, is the true recipe for well-being. So, let's demystify the superfood hype and embrace a realistic, science-backed perspective on nutrition.

Chapter 6

National and International Dietary Guidelines and Recommendations

Tailoring Recommendations for the Indian Market

Dietary guidelines serve as invaluable tools to promote public health, providing evidence-based recommendations for individuals and populations. While global guidelines offer a foundation, it is crucial to tailor these recommendations to the unique dietary habits and preferences of specific regions, such as the diverse and culturally rich Indian market. Here's an overview of both national and international dietary guidelines, adapted to suit the Indian context:

International Guidelines

1. The Mediterranean Diet:

Recommendation: Emphasizes a high intake of fruits, vegetables, nuts, legumes, and whole grains, along with moderate consumption of fish, poultry, and dairy.

Adaptation for India: Incorporate local grains like millets, diverse lentils, and a variety of regional vegetables into the dietary framework.

2. DASH (Dietary Approaches to Stop Hypertension):

Recommendation: Encourages the consumption of fruits, vegetables, whole grains, and lean proteins, and limits sodium intake to manage blood pressure.

Adaptation for India: Include traditional spices like turmeric and cumin for flavoring, and promote the consumption of potassium-rich foods like bananas, citrus fruits, and leafy greens.

National Guidelines:

1. Indian Council of Medical Research (ICMR) Guidelines:

Recommendation: Advocates a balanced diet with an emphasis on locally available foods, including cereals, millets, pulses, fruits, vegetables, milk, and meat.

Adaptation for India: Promote the consumption of traditional grains like ragi, bajra, and jowar alongside popular choices like rice and wheat.

2. Ayurveda-Based Guidelines:

Recommendation: Focuses on balancing doshas (individual constitutions) with an emphasis on seasonal and locally available foods.

Adaptation for India: Incorporate Ayurvedic principles into dietary choices, such as using ghee, turmeric, and ginger in cooking, and consume seasonal fruits and vegetables.

Other Recommendations for the Indian Market:

1. Diverse Plant-Based Diets:

Recommendation: Encourage the consumption of a variety of locally grown fruits, vegetables, and plant-based proteins like lentils and legumes.

Adaptation for India: Highlight the rich diversity of Indian vegetarian cuisine, including regional specialties and incorporating a range of pulses.

2. Inclusion of Healthy Fats:

Recommendation: Promote the consumption of healthy fats such as those found in nuts, seeds, and oily fish.

Adaptation for India: Integrate sources of healthy fats from Indian cuisine, such as almonds, walnuts, sesame seeds, and fish like mackerel.

3. Customizing Portion Sizes:

Recommendation: Provide guidance on portion control to prevent overeating.

Adaptation for India: Consider traditional Indian thali-style meals as a model for balanced portions, incorporating small servings of different dishes.

4. Hydration:

Recommendation: Encourage adequate water intake throughout the day.

Adaptation for India: Recognize the importance of hydrating with water, but also consider traditional hydrating beverages like coconut water and buttermilk.

5. Cultural Sensitivity:

Recommendation: Promote dietary choices that respect cultural and religious preferences.

Adaptation for India: Recognize the diverse dietary practices across regions and communities, respecting the cultural significance of certain foods.

In summary, harmonizing international and national dietary guidelines with the nuances of the Indian market involves celebrating the richness of local cuisines, promoting traditional foods, and respecting cultural preferences. Tailoring recommendations to align with the diverse dietary landscape of India ensures that dietary guidelines are not just informative but also practical and applicable to the daily lives of individuals in this culturally vibrant nation.

Customizing Diets for Individuals

In the realm of nutrition, one size does not fit all. The recognition that each person is unique, with distinct physiological and lifestyle factors, has led to a paradigm shift in dietary recommendations. Customizing diets for individuals is emerging as a cornerstone of promoting health, addressing specific needs, and fostering sustainable well-being. Let's delve into the profound importance of tailoring diets to individual requirements.

1. Acknowledging Bioindividuality:

Every individual possesses a distinct genetic makeup, metabolism, and response to food. What works optimally for one person may not necessarily yield the same results for another. Customizing diets acknowledges and respects this bioindividuality, paving the way for personalized nutrition strategies.

2. Targeting Specific Health Goals:

Customized diets enable individuals to align their eating habits with specific health goals. Whether the aim is weight management, improved energy levels, or managing chronic conditions, tailoring dietary choices ensures that nutritional plans are designed to address individual health aspirations effectively.

3. Catering to Dietary Preferences and Restrictions:

Preferences, allergies, and ethical choices play a significant role in shaping an individual's dietary habits. Customization allows for the incorporation of foods that align with personal preferences while respecting dietary restrictions, making the journey toward health more enjoyable and sustainable.

4. Managing Medical Conditions:

For individuals with specific medical conditions or nutritional requirements, customization is paramount. Conditions like diabetes, celiac disease, or lactose intolerance necessitate tailored dietary plans to manage symptoms, promote healing, and prevent the exacerbation of health issues.

5. Optimizing Nutrient Absorption:

The way individuals absorb and utilize nutrients can vary significantly. Customized diets take into account factors such as gut health, enzyme levels, and nutrient absorption efficiency, ensuring that the chosen foods enhance rather than hinder nutrient utilization.

6. Adapting to Lifestyle Factors:

Lifestyles vary widely, from sedentary office work to physically demanding jobs. Customizing diets involves considering energy expenditure, activity levels, and the demands of daily life. An individualized approach ensures that the diet complements the individual's lifestyle, promoting sustained energy and vitality.

7. Enhancing Mental Well-Being:

The relationship between diet and mental health is intricate. Customizing diets for individuals can include considerations for foods that positively impact mood, cognitive function, and overall mental well-being. This holistic approach recognizes the intricate connection between nutrition and mental health.

8. Encouraging Sustainable Habits:

A diet tailored to an individual's preferences and needs is more likely to be sustainable in the long run. Customization empowers individuals to make choices that resonate with their tastes and lifestyle, fostering a positive relationship with food and promoting adherence to healthy eating patterns.

9. Cultivating a Mindful Approach:

Customized diets encourage mindfulness in eating. By paying attention to individual responses to different foods, individuals can develop a heightened awareness of their body's signals, fostering a mindful and intuitive approach to eating.

10. Respecting Cultural and Culinary Diversity:

Customization respects the richness of cultural and culinary diversity. It acknowledges that dietary patterns are deeply rooted in cultural practices and traditions. By integrating traditional foods and cooking methods, customization ensures that dietary choices align with cultural values.

The importance of customizing diets for individuals transcends the conventional approach of generic dietary recommendations. Recognizing and embracing individual differences in genetics, health goals, lifestyle, and preferences is a pivotal step toward unlocking the full potential of nutrition in promoting optimal health and well-being. Customized diets are not just about what we eat but about crafting a personalized roadmap to wellness that is sustainable, enjoyable, and uniquely tailored to each individual's journey.

Adapting to Cultural and Regional Variations

Embracing Diversity: The Profound Importance of Adapting to Cultural and Regional Variations in Diets

In a world as diverse as ours, where cultures and traditions intermingle to create a rich fabric of identity, the significance of adapting diets to cultural and regional variations cannot be overstated. Nutrition is not a one-size-fits-all concept; rather, it should reflect the diverse culinary landscapes that shape the way we eat. Let's delve into the profound importance of embracing cultural and regional variations in diets.

Preserving Culinary Heritage:

Cultural and regional diets are often rooted in centuries-old traditions, reflecting the unique culinary heritage of communities. Adapting to these variations is a means of preserving and celebrating the authenticity of diverse cuisines, passing down flavors and cooking techniques through generations.

Nutrient-Rich Local Produce:

Different regions boast a variety of local produce that thrives in specific climates. Adapting diets to incorporate these region-specific fruits, vegetables, and grains ensures that individuals benefit from the nutrient richness of locally sourced, seasonal foods, promoting optimal health.

Respecting Dietary Preferences:

Cultural and regional diets respect individual dietary preferences and ethical choices. Whether it's embracing vegetarianism, avoiding specific allergens, or adhering to religious dietary guidelines, adapting diets to cultural variations allows for flexibility while honoring personal choices.

Enhancing Nutritional Balance:

Regional diets are often crafted based on the availability of local ingredients, providing a balanced mix of nutrients suited to the needs of the community. Adapting to these variations ensures that diets are nutritionally comprehensive, addressing the unique health requirements of individuals in different regions.

Promoting Sustainable Eating:

Cultural and regional diets are inherently tied to the local ecosystem. Adapting diets to incorporate sustainable practices, such as consuming locally sourced and seasonal foods, minimizes the environmental impact and promotes eco-friendly eating habits that align with regional sustainability practices.

Cultural Significance of Meals:

Meals are not just about sustenance; they are woven into the fabric of cultural traditions and social rituals. Adapting to cultural variations in diets allows individuals to partake in the shared experience of communal dining, fostering a sense of belonging and connection within communities.

Celebrating Culinary Diversity:

Each culture brings a unique flavor profile to the global culinary tapestry. Adapting to cultural variations celebrates this diversity, inviting individuals to explore and savor a wide array of tastes, textures, and aromas that contribute to the global mosaic of flavors.

Customizing to Health Goals:

Cultural and regional diets can be adapted to align with individual health goals. Whether aiming for weight management, heart health, or other wellness objectives, incorporating region-specific foods and dietary practices offers a personalized approach to health and nutrition.

Preserving Traditional Cooking Methods:

Cultural and regional diets often come with distinct cooking methods that enhance the nutritional value of foods. Adapting to these variations means preserving traditional culinary techniques that contribute to the unique character of regional cuisines.

Fostering Culinary Exploration:

Adapting to cultural and regional variations encourages individuals to embark on culinary explorations, trying new foods and recipes that expand their gastronomic horizons. This sense of culinary adventure adds a layer of excitement to the journey of discovering diverse flavors.

In conclusion, the importance of adapting to cultural and regional variations in diets extends beyond the realm of nutrition. It is a celebration of diversity, a preservation of heritage, and a respectful acknowledgment of the intricate connection between food and culture. By embracing the richness of cultural and regional diets, individuals not only nurture their bodies but also contribute to the collective celebration of global culinary traditions.

Chapter 7

Understanding Food Labels

Decoding Nutritional Information

Navigating the aisles of a grocery store can be overwhelming, especially when faced with an array of food products adorned with nutritional labels. Deciphering the information presented on these labels is crucial for making informed and healthy choices. In this guide, we'll explore how to decode nutritional information on a label, empowering you to make choices that align with your dietary preferences and health goals.

1. Start with Serving Size:

The first step in decoding a nutritional label is understanding the serving size. All the information on the label, including calories and nutrient content, is based on this serving size. Be mindful of portion sizes to accurately assess the nutritional value of what you're consuming.

2. Calories Matter, But They're Not Everything:

Pay attention to the calorie count per serving. However, it's equally important to consider the source of those calories. Nutrient-dense foods with essential vitamins and minerals offer more nutritional value than empty-calorie options.

3. Check the Macronutrients:

Protein: Look for a balance between protein, carbohydrates, and fats. Protein is crucial for muscle repair and overall body function.

Carbohydrates: Consider the type of carbohydrates—favor whole grains over refined sugars. Fiber content is also essential for digestive health.

Fats: Choose products with healthier fats, such as unsaturated fats, and limit saturated and trans fats.

4. Be Mindful of Added Sugars:

Identify the amount of added sugars in the product. Opt for foods with a lower added sugar content, as excessive sugar intake is linked to various health issues. Keep in mind that natural sugars in fruits and dairy are not the same as added sugars.

5. Fiber is Your Friend:

Adequate fiber intake is crucial for digestive health and can contribute to a feeling of fullness. Foods high in fiber are generally more nutritious and can help regulate blood sugar levels.

6. Watch Out for Sodium:

Keep an eye on the sodium content, especially if you're managing your blood pressure. High sodium intake is associated with an increased risk of hypertension and cardiovascular issues.

7. Understand Percent Daily Values (%DV):

Percent Daily Values on the label indicate how much a nutrient in a serving contributes to a daily diet. Use %DV as a rough guide—aim for nutrients like fiber, vitamins, and minerals to be closer to 100% and limit those like saturated fats and sodium.

8. Look Beyond the Front Label:

Don't rely solely on front-of-package claims like "low-fat" or "all-natural." Flip the product and scrutinize the detailed nutritional information to get a comprehensive understanding.

9. Consider Allergen Information:

If you have allergies or sensitivities, review the allergen information. Food labels are required to highlight common allergens like nuts, dairy, soy, and gluten.

10. Ingredient List Matters:

The ingredient list provides insight into the quality of the product. Ingredients are listed in descending order by weight, so the first few ingredients are the most prominent. Choose products with a shorter and more recognizable ingredient list.

11. Watch Out for Serving Tricks:

Some products may appear to have a low calorie or sugar content, but the serving size might be tiny. Be mindful of portion sizes to get an accurate picture of what you're consuming.

12. Compare Products:

When in doubt, compare similar products. Choose the one with better nutritional value and fewer additives.

Decoding nutritional information on food labels is an essential skill for making informed dietary choices. By understanding serving sizes, paying attention to macronutrients, and being mindful of added sugars and other key components, you can empower yourself to make healthier decisions at the grocery store. Remember, a little extra time spent reading labels can go a long way toward supporting your overall well-being.

Spotting Hidden Sugars and Additives

Navigating the aisles of a grocery store can feel like deciphering a secret code when it comes to identifying hidden sugars and additives in food labels. Many seemingly healthy products can hide sweeteners and other not-so-beneficial ingredients. This guide aims to empower you to unveil these hidden culprits, allowing you to make informed choices that align with your health goals.

1. Beware of Sugar Aliases:

Spotting Hidden Sugars: Manufacturers often use various names for sugar to make it less obvious. Look for terms like sucrose, high-fructose corn syrup, agave nectar, and other syrupy aliases. If a product has multiple sugar sources listed, it likely contains hidden sugars.

2. Check the Ingredient List:

Position Matters: Ingredients are listed in descending order by weight. If sugar or a sweetener is among the first few ingredients, it's a sign that the product is high in added sugars.

Hidden Names: Apart from direct references to sugar, watch out for terms like maltose, dextrose, fructose, and other sweetening agents.

3. Watch for Artificial Sweeteners:

Look Beyond "Sugar-Free": Products labeled as "sugar-free" may contain artificial sweeteners. Common ones include aspartame, saccharin, and sucralose. Be cautious if you're sensitive to or prefer to avoid these additives.

4. Sneaky Sugars in Savory Products:

Sauces and Condiments: Salad dressings, ketchup, and other condiments can harbor hidden sugars. Check the ingredient list for sweeteners in these savory items.

Low-Fat Products: Reduced-fat or fat-free products often compensate for flavor by adding sugar. Scrutinize labels to ensure the reduction in fat doesn't translate to an increase in sugars.

5. Crack the Code of Code Words:

Natural vs. Added: Not all sugars are created equal. Natural sugars found in fruits and dairy come with fiber and nutrients. Added sugars, on the other hand, contribute to empty calories. Distinguish between the two for a more nuanced understanding.

6. Identify Hidden Additives:

Preservatives: Scan for additives and preservatives in the ingredient list. Words like BHA, BHT, and sodium benzoate may indicate the presence of additives.

Colorings and Flavorings: Artificial colorings and flavorings may be lurking in processed foods. Look for specific color names and terms like "artificial flavor."

7. Check for Whole Grains:

Whole vs. Refined Grains: Products labeled as "whole grain" may still contain hidden sugars. Check for refined grains, as they can contribute to elevated sugar content.

8. Be Mindful of Serving Sizes:

Calculated Sugars: Be mindful of serving sizes when evaluating sugar content. A seemingly low-sugar product may become a significant source if consumed in larger quantities.

9. Be Wary of Health Claims:

Misleading Claims: Products labeled as "healthy" or "natural" can still contain hidden sugars. Rely on the ingredient list rather than front-of-package claims.

10. Educate Yourself on Common Additives:

Research Ingredients: Familiarize yourself with common additives and sweeteners. This knowledge empowers you to make more informed decisions when faced with unfamiliar ingredients.

Decoding food labels to spot hidden sugars and additives requires a keen eye and a bit of nutritional detective work. By carefully examining ingredient lists, understanding sugar aliases, and being mindful of common additives, you can unveil the hidden culprits and make choices that align with your health and wellness goals. Remember, the more you know about what's in your food, the better equipped you are to make healthier choices for you and your family.

Chapter 8

Nutrition and Chronic Diseases

In the contemporary landscape of healthcare, the role of nutrition in preventing chronic diseases has garnered significant attention. As the prevalence of conditions like heart disease, diabetes, and certain cancers continues to rise, understanding the intricate connection between dietary choices and long-term health becomes paramount. This article explores the multifaceted relationship between nutrition and chronic diseases, emphasizing the importance of a holistic approach to well-being.

The Foundation: Building Health through Nutrition:

Heart Health: A heart-healthy diet is characterized by the incorporation of fruits, vegetables, whole grains, and lean proteins. The consumption of omega-3 fatty acids found in fatty fish, flaxseeds, and walnuts has been associated with a reduced risk of cardiovascular diseases.

Diabetes Prevention and Management: Nutrition plays a pivotal role in diabetes prevention and management. Emphasizing complex carbohydrates, fiber-rich foods, and balanced meals helps regulate blood sugar levels. Monitoring portion sizes and choosing nutrient-dense foods are crucial for individuals with diabetes or those at risk.

Cancer Risk Reduction: Certain dietary patterns and food choices have been linked to a lower risk of cancer. A diet rich in antioxidants from colorful fruits and vegetables, along with the inclusion of cruciferous vegetables and whole grains, contributes to a protective effect against various types of cancer.

Bone Health: An adequate intake of calcium and vitamin D is essential for maintaining strong and healthy bones. Dairy products, leafy greens, and exposure to sunlight are valuable sources of these nutrients, contributing to the prevention of osteoporosis.

Nutrition as a Preventive Measure:

Whole Foods vs. Processed Foods: Prioritizing whole, unprocessed foods over highly processed options is key to preventing chronic diseases. Whole foods provide essential nutrients, fiber, and antioxidants, while processed foods often contain added sugars, unhealthy fats, and artificial additives.

Balanced Macronutrients: Achieving a balance of macronutrients—proteins, carbohydrates, and fats—is crucial for overall health. Opting for lean proteins, complex carbohydrates, and healthy fats supports optimal body function and reduces the risk of obesity-related conditions.

Mindful Eating Practices: Adopting mindful eating practices, such as paying attention to hunger and fullness cues, helps prevent overeating. Mindful eating promotes a healthy relationship with food and supports weight management, a critical factor in chronic disease prevention.

The Mediterranean Diet: A Model for Wellness:

The Mediterranean diet serves as a compelling model for promoting overall health and preventing chronic diseases. Rich in fruits, vegetables, whole grains, olive oil, and fish, this dietary pattern provides a wealth of nutrients, healthy fats, and antioxidants associated with a lower risk of heart disease and other chronic conditions.

Educational Initiatives for Nutritional Literacy:

Fostering nutritional literacy is crucial for empowering individuals to make informed dietary choices. Educational initiatives that teach the fundamentals of nutrition, decipher food labels, and provide practical cooking skills can contribute significantly to chronic disease prevention.

Nutrition emerges as a powerful tool in the prevention of chronic diseases, offering a proactive approach to health and well-being. By embracing a diet rich in whole, nutrient-dense foods, individuals can navigate the intricate landscape of chronic disease risk factors. The journey towards a healthier future involves not just understanding the link between nutrition and chronic diseases but actively incorporating sustainable dietary practices into everyday life. It's time to recognize the transformative potential of our food choices in shaping a resilient and thriving tomorrow.

Preventing Heart Disease Through Diet

Heart disease remains a prevalent and serious health concern, but the good news is that adopting a heart-healthy diet can significantly reduce the risk and contribute to overall cardiovascular well-being. In this article, we explore the essential elements of a diet that play a pivotal role in preventing heart disease, offering practical insights for individuals keen on nurturing their heart health.

1. The Power of Plant-Based Foods:

Colorful Fruits and Vegetables: Packed with vitamins, minerals, and antioxidants, fruits and vegetables contribute to heart health by reducing inflammation and supporting overall cardiovascular function.

Whole Grains: Opt for whole grains like oats, brown rice, and quinoa, which provide fiber, aid in cholesterol management, and maintain steady blood sugar levels.

2. Lean Proteins for Heart Health:

Fatty Fish: Fatty fish like salmon, mackerel, and trout are rich in omega-3 fatty acids. These healthy fats have been shown to lower blood pressure, reduce triglycerides, and decrease the risk of abnormal heart rhythms.

Plant-Based Proteins: Incorporate plant-based protein sources such as legumes, beans, and nuts. These alternatives to red and processed meats contribute to a lower saturated fat intake.

3. Healthy Fats for a Happy Heart:

Heart-Healthy Oils: Choose oils rich in monounsaturated and polyunsaturated fats, like olive oil and canola oil. These fats have cardiovascular benefits, including lowering bad cholesterol levels.

Nuts and Seeds: Almonds, walnuts, chia seeds, and flaxseeds are excellent sources of heart-healthy fats, fiber, and antioxidants.

4. Mindful Sodium Management:

Reducing Processed Foods: Limit processed and packaged foods, as they often contain high levels of sodium. Excessive sodium intake is linked to hypertension, a significant risk factor for heart disease.

Herbs and Spices: Flavor meals with herbs and spices instead of excessive salt. This not only enhances taste but also contributes to heart health.

5. Moderate Sugar Intake:

Limit Added Sugar: Excessive sugar intake can contribute to obesity and diabetes, both risk factors for heart disease. Choose whole fruits over sugary snacks and beverages to satisfy sweet cravings.

6. Portion Control and Weight Management:

Balanced Portions: Be mindful of portion sizes to avoid overeating. Maintaining a healthy weight reduces the strain on the heart and lowers the risk of heart disease.

Regular Physical Activity: Combine a heart-healthy diet with regular physical activity to support weight management and overall cardiovascular health.

7. Hydration for Heart Health:

Water as the Primary Beverage: Choose water as the main beverage to stay hydrated without added sugars or calories. Proper hydration supports optimal heart function.

8. Limiting Alcohol Intake:

Moderation is Key: If you consume alcohol, do so in moderation. Excessive alcohol intake can contribute to high blood pressure and increase the risk of heart disease.

9. Regular Checkups and Monitoring:

Blood Pressure and Cholesterol Checks: Regularly monitor blood pressure and cholesterol levels. High blood pressure and elevated cholesterol are significant contributors to heart disease.

10. Consultation with Healthcare Professionals:

Individualized Approaches: Consult healthcare professionals for personalized advice. They can guide dietary choices tailored to individual health conditions and risk factors.

Preventing heart disease through diet is an empowering journey that involves making thoughtful and heart-healthy choices every day. By embracing a diet rich in fruits, vegetables, lean proteins, and healthy fats while minimizing sodium, sugar, and processed foods, individuals can pave the way for a heart-healthy lifestyle. Coupled with regular exercise and attentive healthcare monitoring, these dietary practices contribute to a lifetime of cardiovascular well-being. Remember, each bite is a step toward a healthier heart, and the choices you make in the kitchen can shape a future of heart resilience and vitality.

Managing Diabetes with Nutrition

Living with diabetes necessitates a mindful and proactive approach to nutrition. The choices made in the kitchen play a pivotal role in managing blood sugar levels and promoting overall well-being. In this section, we'll explore the key principles of managing diabetes through nutrition, offering valuable insights for individuals on the journey to balance and control.

1. Embracing a Balanced Plate:

Portion Control: Paying attention to portion sizes helps regulate carbohydrate intake, which directly influences blood sugar levels.

Balanced Macronutrients: Incorporate a mix of carbohydrates, proteins, and healthy fats into each meal for sustained energy and stable blood sugar.

2. Carbohydrate Management:

Focus on Complex Carbs: Opt for complex carbohydrates with a lower glycemic index, such as whole grains, legumes, and vegetables. These choices lead to a slower rise in blood sugar.

Fiber-Rich Foods: High-fiber foods like fruits, vegetables, and whole grains contribute to better blood sugar control and improved digestive health.

3. Smart Protein Choices:

Lean Proteins: Choose lean protein sources like poultry, fish, tofu, and legumes to support muscle health without affecting blood sugar levels.

Plant-Based Proteins: Incorporate plant-based proteins for variety and additional health benefits. Beans, lentils, and nuts are excellent choices.

4. Healthy Fats for Heart Health:

Monounsaturated and Polyunsaturated Fats: Include sources of healthy fats, such as avocados, olive oil, and nuts. These fats support heart health and provide a steady source of energy.

5. Mindful Sugar Management:

Limit Added Sugars: Minimize the consumption of foods and beverages with added sugars. Opt for naturally sweet alternatives like fruits to satisfy sweet cravings.

Read Labels: Scrutinize food labels for hidden sugars and be aware of various names for sugar derivatives.

6. Consistent Meal Timing:

Regular Meals: Establish a routine of regular meals and snacks to maintain stable blood sugar levels throughout the day.

Avoid Skipping Meals: Skipping meals can lead to erratic blood sugar spikes and crashes.

7. Hydration Importance:

Water as the Primary Beverage: Choose water as the main beverage to stay hydrated without affecting blood sugar levels.

Limit Sugary Drinks: Avoid sugary beverages that can lead to rapid increases in blood sugar.

8. Individualized Nutritional Planning:

Consult with a Dietitian: Collaborate with a registered dietitian to create a personalized nutrition plan. Individualized approaches factor in specific dietary needs, preferences, and lifestyle considerations.

9. Monitoring Blood Sugar Levels:

Regular Monitoring: Consistently monitor blood sugar levels to understand how different foods and meals impact individual responses.

Adjust as Needed: Use blood sugar readings to make informed adjustments to dietary choices and insulin or medication dosages.

10. Holistic Lifestyle Integration:

Regular Exercise: Combine a balanced diet with regular physical activity to enhance blood sugar control and overall well-being.

Stress Management: Incorporate stress-reducing practices, as stress can impact blood sugar levels. Techniques like meditation and mindfulness can be beneficial.

Managing diabetes through nutrition is an ongoing journey that requires dedication and mindfulness. By adopting a balanced and individualized approach to dietary choices, individuals can effectively control blood sugar levels and promote overall health. Nutrition becomes not just a means of managing diabetes but a powerful tool for cultivating a lifestyle of well-being, resilience, and vitality. Remember, with each nourishing bite, you contribute to a future of balanced health and diabetes management.

The Impact of Nutrition on Cancer Prevention

The intersection between nutrition and cancer management is a dynamic and evolving field that underscores the significance of dietary choices in supporting both treatment outcomes and overall well-being. In this article, we'll delve into the impact of nutrition in cancer management, exploring how a thoughtful approach to diet can play a pivotal role in enhancing the quality of life for individuals on the cancer journey.

1. Sustaining Strength and Energy:

Protein-Rich Foods: Adequate protein intake is essential for maintaining muscle mass and strength, especially during cancer treatments. Lean meats, poultry, fish, and plant-based sources like beans and lentils are valuable choices.

Complex Carbohydrates: Whole grains, fruits, and vegetables provide a sustained source of energy, which is crucial for individuals undergoing cancer therapies that may lead to fatigue.

2. Managing Treatment Side Effects:

Nausea and Digestive Issues: Ginger, peppermint, and easily digestible foods can help manage nausea and digestive discomfort commonly associated with cancer treatments.

Hydration: Staying hydrated is vital to managing dehydration caused by treatments like chemotherapy. Water, herbal teas, and hydrating foods like fruits contribute to fluid intake.

3. Immune System Support:

Antioxidant-Rich Foods: Fruits and vegetables rich in antioxidants, such as berries, leafy greens, and citrus fruits, support the immune system and help combat oxidative stress.

Zinc and Selenium: Foods containing zinc (pumpkin seeds, chickpeas) and selenium (Brazil nuts, fish) contribute to immune function.

4. Weight Management and Nutrient Density:

Maintaining a Healthy Weight: Adequate caloric intake is crucial for preventing unintentional weight loss, a common concern during cancer treatment. Nutrient-dense foods provide essential vitamins and minerals without excess calories.

Healthy Fats: Incorporate sources of healthy fats, such as avocados, nuts, and olive oil, to support overall nutrition and caloric intake.

5. Hydration for Well-being:

Balanced Fluid Intake: Proper hydration is essential for overall health and can help manage side effects like dry mouth and difficulty swallowing. Encourage a balance of water, herbal teas, and hydrating foods.

6. Individualized Nutrition Plans:

Consultation with a Dietitian: Collaborate with a registered dietitian who specializes in oncology to create a personalized nutrition plan. Individualized approaches consider specific treatment regimens, nutritional needs, and preferences.

7. Maintaining Nutrient Balance:

Proper Nutrient Ratios: Balance macronutrients, ensuring a mix of carbohydrates, proteins, and fats. This supports overall nutritional balance and addresses the unique needs of cancer patients.

8. Mindful Eating Practices:

Listening to Body Signals: Encourage mindful eating practices to listen to hunger and fullness cues. This can be particularly helpful for individuals experiencing changes in appetite during treatment.

9. Addressing Taste Changes:

Flavorful Options: Experiment with herbs and spices to add flavor to meals for individuals experiencing taste changes or a loss of appetite.

Small, Frequent Meals: Offering smaller, more frequent meals can be more manageable for those dealing with changes in taste.

10. Supporting Emotional Well-being:

Community and Social Support: Encourage a supportive community and social environment around meals. Emotional well-being is intertwined with nutritional health during the cancer journey.

The impact of nutrition in cancer management extends far beyond sustaining physical health; it encompasses a holistic approach to overall well-being. By embracing thoughtful dietary choices tailored to individual needs, individuals navigating cancer treatments can optimize their nutritional status, manage treatment side effects, and enhance their quality of life. Nutrition becomes a powerful ally in the fight against cancer, supporting resilience, strength, and a sense of empowerment throughout the cancer journey.

Chapter 9

Sports Nutrition and Performance

Sports nutrition stands as a cornerstone in the realm of athletic performance, wielding a profound influence on the outcomes achieved by athletes. Beyond the physical exertion on the field, track, or court, the choices made in the kitchen become paramount in determining the success and endurance of individuals engaged in sports. Optimal energy levels, a prerequisite for any athlete, are sustained through a strategic intake of carbohydrates, the primary source of fuel for the body. Proteins, pivotal for muscle support and repair, play a crucial role in the development and maintenance of an athlete's physical prowess. Hydration, often underestimated, is the linchpin for optimal performance, ensuring proper fluid balance, electrolyte replacement, and a reduction in the risk of cramping. Micronutrients, encompassing vitamins and minerals, contribute not only to overall health but also to the intricate processes vital for athletic excellence. Sports nutrition extends its impact on weight management, body composition goals, and the timing and frequency of meals, offering a comprehensive approach to fueling athletic achievements. Moreover, it emphasizes the importance of gut health, immune system support, and mental focus, recognizing that peak performance transcends the physical to encompass holistic well-being. In essence, sports nutrition serves as the unsung hero, working behind the scenes to fortify athletes on their journey to success, ensuring that every stride, sprint, or swing is fueled by the optimal combination of nutrients and strategic dietary choices.

Fueling Your Body for Exercise

Embarking on an exercise journey requires more than just enthusiasm; it demands a strategic approach to fueling your body for optimal performance and recovery. The right combination of nutrients can be the difference between a lackluster workout and one that leaves you feeling energized and accomplished. In this article, we'll delve into the art and science of smart nutrition to fuel your body for exercise.

1. Pre-Workout Nutrition: Setting the Stage for Success:

Before lacing up your sneakers, consider a pre-workout nutrition strategy. Carbohydrates take center stage here, providing a readily available energy source. Opt for complex carbs like whole grains and fruits for sustained energy release during your workout. Pairing carbohydrates with a moderate amount of protein can enhance endurance and muscle support.

2. Hydration: The Foundation of Peak Performance:

Hydration is a non-negotiable aspect of effective exercise fueling. Dehydration can lead to fatigue, cramping, and compromised performance. Ensure you're well hydrated before, during, and after your workout. Water is a reliable choice, but for longer and more intense sessions, consider sports drinks that replenish electrolytes lost through sweat.

3. Intra-Workout Nutrition: Maintaining Momentum:

For prolonged workouts, especially those exceeding an hour, consider intra-workout nutrition to maintain energy levels. This can involve consuming easily digestible carbohydrates, such as energy gels or sports drinks, to replenish glycogen stores and stave off fatigue. Tailor your choices based on the duration and intensity of your exercise.

4. Post-Workout Recovery: Repair and Refuel:

The post-workout window is a critical period for recovery and replenishment. Protein plays a key role here, aiding in muscle repair and growth. Pairing protein with carbohydrates enhances glycogen replenishment. Foods like lean chicken, Greek yogurt, or a protein smoothie with fruits can be excellent choices.

5. Protein-Packed Power: Building Blocks of Strength:

Protein is a cornerstone of exercise nutrition, serving as the building block for muscle tissue. Include a variety of protein sources in your diet, such as lean meats, poultry, fish, eggs, dairy, legumes, and plant-based options like tofu and tempeh. Aim for a balanced distribution of protein throughout the day to support ongoing muscle maintenance.

6. Healthy Fats: A Sustained Energy Source:

While carbohydrates take the lead in providing quick energy, healthy fats play a role in sustaining endurance. Include sources of monounsaturated and polyunsaturated fats in your diet, such as avocados, nuts, seeds, and olive oil. These fats contribute to overall energy balance and support long-duration activities.

7. Timing is Key: Tailoring Nutrition to Your Schedule:

Consider the timing of your meals and snacks in relation to your exercise routine. Eating a balanced meal 2-3 hours before exercise allows for proper digestion, while a small snack 30-60 minutes before can provide a quick energy boost. Post-workout nutrition should be consumed within the first hour after exercise to optimize recovery.

8. Individualized Approaches: Listen to Your Body:

Every individual is unique, and so are their nutritional needs. Listen to your body's signals and adjust your nutrition plan accordingly. Factors such as the type of exercise, intensity, and personal tolerance play a role in determining what works best for you.

9. Balancing Macronutrients: A Holistic Approach:

A holistic approach to exercise nutrition involves balancing macronutrients—carbohydrates, proteins, and fats. Each macronutrient plays a specific role in supporting energy, muscle function, and overall health. Customize your macronutrient distribution based on your fitness goals and the nature of your workouts.

10. Consistency and Sustainability: Building Habits for the Long Run:

Effective exercise nutrition is not a one-time effort; it's about building sustainable habits. Consistency in nourishing your body with the right nutrients, staying hydrated, and adapting your plan as needed contribute to long-term success in achieving fitness goals.

Fueling your body for exercise is a dynamic and personalized journey that integrates science and strategy. By understanding the nuances of pre-workout, intra-workout, and post-workout nutrition and making thoughtful choices about macronutrients, hydration, and timing, you empower yourself to achieve peak performance and support overall well-being. Whether you're hitting the gym, pounding the pavement, or flowing through a yoga session, let your nutrition be the ally that propels you toward your fitness aspirations.

Hydration Strategies

Optimizing Performance: Hydration Strategies in Sports Nutrition

Hydration stands as a linchpin in the realm of sports nutrition, wielding a profound impact on athletic performance, endurance, and recovery. The strategic management of fluids becomes pivotal, not just to quench thirst but to sustain peak physical function. Let's take a look at effective hydration strategies that athletes can integrate into their sports nutrition regimen for optimal results.

1. Pre-Hydration: Starting Strong:

The foundation for effective hydration begins before the workout or competition. Athletes should aim to start well-hydrated by consuming fluids throughout the day leading up to their activity. Water is a fundamental choice, but for prolonged and intense efforts, electrolyte-rich sports drinks can be beneficial in maintaining proper fluid and electrolyte balance.

2. Individualized Hydration Plans: Recognizing Unique Needs:

No two athletes are the same, and hydration needs can vary based on factors such as body weight, activity intensity, and environmental conditions. Establishing an individualized hydration plan that considers these factors is crucial. Athletes can work with sports nutrition professionals to tailor hydration strategies to their specific requirements.

3. Hydration Monitoring: Beyond Thirst Quenching:

While thirst is a reliable indicator of dehydration, relying solely on this sensation may lead to suboptimal performance. Athletes should adopt proactive hydration monitoring methods, such as assessing urine color or using sweat rate calculations. These tools provide valuable insights into fluid balance and guide timely hydration adjustments.

4. Electrolyte Considerations: Balancing More than Water:

Intense physical activity results in the loss of electrolytes through sweat. Sodium, potassium, and other electrolytes play crucial roles in muscle function and nerve impulses. Hydration strategies should encompass replenishing these essential minerals, either through balanced meals or electrolyte-rich beverages.

5. Timing Matters: Strategic Hydration Throughout:

Effective hydration is not a one-time effort; it's a continuous process throughout the activity. Athletes should develop a habit of sipping fluids regularly, aiming for a steady intake rather than large volumes at once. This approach helps maintain optimal hydration levels and minimizes the risk of dehydration.

6. Hydration During Exercise: Choosing the Right Fluids:

The choice of fluids during exercise is pivotal. Water remains a fundamental option, but for prolonged activities lasting more than an hour, sports drinks containing carbohydrates and electrolytes can offer additional benefits. These beverages contribute to maintaining energy levels and preventing electrolyte imbalances.

7. Post-Exercise Rehydration: Closing the Hydration Loop:

The post-exercise period is a critical window for rehydration and recovery. Athletes should prioritize replenishing fluids lost during the activity. Including a mix of water, sports drinks, and recovery beverages with protein can aid in restoring hydration levels and kickstart the recovery process.

8. Weather and Environmental Factors: Adapting to Conditions:

Environmental conditions, such as heat and humidity, significantly impact fluid requirements. Athletes should adapt their hydration strategies based on weather forecasts and activity conditions. In hot and humid environments, increased fluid intake and attention to electrolyte balance become even more crucial.

9. Hydration and Weight Management: Balancing Act:

Athletes often focus on maintaining optimal body weight, but drastic fluid restriction for weight loss can compromise performance and health. Effective hydration strategies align with weight management goals, emphasizing the importance of gradual and sustainable practices.

10. Educational Initiatives: Empowering Athletes:

Promoting awareness and education on hydration within sports teams and organizations is essential. Athletes benefit from understanding the science behind hydration, recognizing their unique needs, and implementing evidence-based strategies. Hydration education fosters a proactive approach among athletes toward optimizing their performance.

Hydration strategies in sports nutrition go beyond simply drinking water; they encompass a nuanced and individualized approach to fluid management. Athletes who integrate these strategies into their training and competition routines gain a competitive edge, ensuring they are well-fueled, resilient, and primed for peak performance. By recognizing the multifaceted nature of hydration and adopting proactive measures, athletes can harness the power of optimal fluid balance to propel themselves toward success on the field, track, or court.

Pre and Post-Workout Nutrition

Unveiling the Power of Pre- and Post-Workout Nutrition: Elevating Your Fitness Game

Embarking on a fitness journey requires more than just breaking a sweat; it necessitates a strategic approach to nutrition that optimally fuels your body for the demands of exercise and aids in efficient recovery. The importance of pre- and post-workout nutrition cannot be overstated, as these windows offer unique opportunities to enhance performance, support energy levels, and promote muscle recovery.

Pre-workout nutrition serves as the key to unlocking your body's potential, ensuring that it is adequately fueled for the upcoming physical exertion. Consider the following components:

1. Carbohydrates as Fuel:

Energy Reserves: Consuming complex carbohydrates before a workout provides a sustainable source of energy. Opt for whole grains, fruits, and vegetables to fuel your muscles and prevent early fatigue.

2. Protein for Muscle Support:

Preventing Muscle Breakdown: Including a moderate amount of protein in your pre-workout meal or snack aids in preventing muscle breakdown during exercise. Lean protein sources such as poultry, fish, or plant-based alternatives are excellent choices.

3. Hydration Matters:

Preventing Dehydration: Adequate hydration before exercise is crucial for optimal performance. Start your workout well-hydrated by sipping water throughout the day, and consider a sports drink if your session is particularly intense or prolonged.

4. Timing is Everything:

Balanced Timing: Consume your pre-workout meal or snack about 2-3 hours before exercising to allow for proper digestion. If you have less time, opt for a smaller snack 30-60 minutes before your workout.

Post-Workout Nutrition: Nourishing Your Body for Recovery

Post-workout nutrition is the cornerstone of efficient recovery, helping your body repair and replenish after the physical demands of exercise. Consider the following elements:

1. Protein for Muscle Repair:

Muscle Recovery: Post-exercise, the body enters a phase of heightened protein synthesis. Consuming a protein-rich meal or snack within the first hour helps kickstart the muscle repair process. Opt for sources like eggs, yogurt, or a protein shake.

2. Carbohydrates for Glycogen Replenishment:

Restoring Energy Stores: Replenishing glycogen stores, depleted during exercise, is vital for sustained energy levels. Consuming carbohydrates alongside protein enhances glycogen replenishment. Choose whole grains, fruits, or sweet potatoes.

3. Hydration for Recovery:

Rehydrating after Sweat Loss: Rehydration is a crucial aspect of post-workout nutrition. Replace fluids lost through sweat by consuming water or a sports drink, especially if your workout was intense or in hot conditions.

4. Nutrient-Dense Choices:

Essential Nutrients: Post-workout meals should be nutrient-dense, providing a mix of vitamins, minerals, and antioxidants. Include a variety of colorful fruits and vegetables to support overall health.

5. Balancing Macronutrients:

Comprehensive Nutrition: A balanced post-workout meal includes a combination of carbohydrates, proteins, and healthy fats. This combination promotes optimal recovery and supports various physiological processes.

Harmonizing Pre- and Post-Workout Nutrition

The synergy between pre- and post-workout nutrition creates a harmonious balance that optimizes your fitness endeavors. Pre-workout nutrition ensures your body is primed for action, maximizing energy stores and preventing premature fatigue. Post-workout nutrition swoops in to replenish what was expended, fostering muscle recovery and setting the stage for future gains.

In conclusion, the importance of pre- and post-workout nutrition lies in their ability to act as catalysts for success on your fitness journey. By understanding the unique roles each plays and tailoring your nutrition to your exercise routine, you unlock the full potential of your body, ensuring that every rep, run, or yoga session is a step toward your wellness goals.

Importance of Protein in Muscle Building

Protein's Crucial Role in Muscle Building: A Foundation for Fitness Success

When it comes to sculpting a strong and resilient physique, protein is the hero-nutrient in the world of nutrition. The importance of protein in muscle building cannot be overstated; it serves as the fundamental building block that fuels growth, repair, and overall strength. In this article, we delve into the critical role of protein in the process of muscle building and why it stands as an indispensable component of any successful fitness regimen.

1. Muscle Protein Synthesis: The Key to Growth:

Anabolism in Action: Protein is rich in amino acids, the essential components that drive muscle protein synthesis—the process by which new muscle tissue is formed. Adequate protein intake provides the raw materials necessary for the body to build and repair muscle.

2. Supporting Lean Muscle Mass:

Preserving and Building: Protein plays a pivotal role in both preserving existing muscle mass and fostering the development of new muscle tissue. This is particularly crucial for individuals engaged in resistance training or those seeking to enhance their overall strength.

3. Optimizing Workout Recovery:

Repair and Regeneration: Intense exercise leads to micro-tears in muscle fibers. Protein steps in as the repair crew, aiding in the regeneration of damaged tissues. Consuming protein post-workout enhances recovery, ensuring you're ready for the next training session.

4. Protein's Thermogenic Effect:

Boosting Metabolism: Protein has a higher thermogenic effect compared to fats and carbohydrates. This means the body expends more energy (calories) to digest and process protein. This metabolic boost can contribute to weight management and fat loss while promoting muscle development.

5. Satiety and Weight Management:

Curbing Hunger: Protein-rich meals induce a feeling of satiety, helping to control hunger and prevent overeating. This characteristic is particularly beneficial for those aiming to manage their body weight while striving to build and maintain muscle mass.

6. Optimizing Nutrient Timing:

Strategic Consumption: Timing matters when it comes to protein intake. Consuming protein-rich meals or snacks around the time of your workout, especially post-exercise, enhances the body's ability to utilize amino acids for muscle repair and growth.

7. Variety for Comprehensive Nutrition:

Diverse Sources: Including a variety of protein sources in your diet ensures you receive a spectrum of essential amino acids. Animal sources like lean meats, poultry, fish, dairy, and plant-based sources like legumes, tofu, and quinoa contribute to a well-rounded protein intake.

8. Individualized Protein Needs:

Tailoring Intake: Protein requirements vary based on factors such as age, gender, activity level, and fitness goals. Tailoring your protein intake to meet your specific needs ensures you provide your body with the right amount for optimal muscle building without excess.

9. Consistency for Long-Term Gains:

Sustainable Habits: The key to successful muscle building lies in consistency. Establishing sustainable habits of incorporating protein into your daily meals and snacks sets the stage for long-term gains and overall fitness success.

10. Balancing Macronutrients:

Holistic Nutrition: Protein works synergistically with other macronutrients—carbohydrates and fats. A balanced intake of these macronutrients supports overall energy needs, allowing the protein to focus on its primary role in muscle building.

Protein assumes the role of the master weaver in the complex design of the human body, intricately crafting its strength and resilience. From fueling muscle protein synthesis to aiding in recovery and promoting satiety, protein stands as the cornerstone of any effective muscle-building endeavor. Recognizing the importance of protein and integrating it strategically into your nutrition plan ensures that every rep, set, and workout contributes to the sculpting of a powerful and enduring physique.

Chapter 10

Eating for Mental Health

Nourishing the Mind and Understanding the Intricate Connection Between Nutrition and Mental Health

In the pursuit of holistic well-being, the impact of nutrition on mental health has emerged as a pivotal and multifaceted aspect. Beyond its role in physical health, the food we consume plays a significant role in shaping cognitive function, emotional resilience, and overall mental wellness. The symbiotic relationship between the gut and the brain, known as the gut-brain axis, underscores the significance of a well-nourished digestive system in promoting mental well-being. Research increasingly highlights the role of specific nutrients in the synthesis of neurotransmitters—chemical messengers crucial for mood regulation. Omega-3 fatty acids, found in abundance in fatty fish, exemplify how dietary choices can directly contribute to the production of serotonin, a neurotransmitter associated with happiness and emotional balance.

The delicate balance between blood sugar and mood stability is a complicated relationship that highlights the need of selecting complex carbs that offer long-lasting energy and mental clarity. Antioxidants, abundant in fruits, vegetables, and nuts, act as guardians of brain health, combating oxidative stress associated with mental health disorders. Probiotics, present in fermented foods like yogurt, contribute to a healthy gut microbiome, influencing mental well-being. Mindful eating practices, emphasizing the sensory aspects of consuming food, foster a positive relationship with nutrition and reduce stress.

Hydration, often overlooked in discussions about mental health, is fundamental for clear thinking and optimal cognitive function. The choice between whole foods and highly processed options is critical, with the former providing essential nutrients and the latter potentially contributing to inflammation and negative mental health outcomes. A balanced, comprehensive approach to nutrition is essential for maintaining a diverse, high-nutrient diet that promotes general well-being.

In the area of mental health, individualization or customization is key. Seeking professional guidance from registered dietitians or nutrition experts allows for the customization of nutrition plans to address specific needs, complementing other therapeutic measures. As our understanding of the intricate connection between nutrition and mental health deepens, embracing a conscious and intentional approach to eating emerges as a tangible and accessible means of fostering not only physical vitality but also the resilience and vibrancy of the mind. It is a journey toward nourishing not just the body, but also the complete web of thoughts and emotions that collectively define our mental landscape.

The Gut-Brain Connection

Understanding the Gut-Brain Connection

Within the complicated structure of the human body, an important conversation takes place between the brain and the gut; this dynamic exchange extends beyond the context of digestion to include all aspects of mental health and general well-being. This intricate connection, known as the gut-brain connection or gut-brain axis, has become a focal point of scientific exploration, revealing a profound interplay between the gut, the nervous system, and the mind.

At the heart of this connection lies the enteric nervous system, often referred to as the "second brain," which comprises a complex network of neurons embedded in the walls of the gastrointestinal tract. This "second brain" communicates with the central nervous system through an extensive network of neural pathways, hormones, and immune system mediators.

1. Communicating Through Neurotransmitters:

The gut and the brain communicate using neurotransmitters, the chemical messengers that transmit signals between nerve cells. Serotonin, a neurotransmitter traditionally associated with mood regulation, is primarily produced in the gut. This sheds light on the impact of gut health on emotional well-being.

2. Microbiota Matters:

The gut is home to trillions of microorganisms, collectively known as the gut microbiota. This diverse community of bacteria, viruses, and fungi not only aids in digestion but also plays a crucial role in influencing the gut-brain connection.

Emerging research suggests that the composition of the microbiota can impact mood, stress responses, and cognitive function.

3. Influence on Mental Health:

Imbalances in the gut microbiota have been linked to various mental health conditions, including anxiety, depression, and even neurodegenerative diseases. The bidirectional communication between the gut and the brain means that mental health can influence gut health and vice versa.

4. Stress Response and the Gut:

The gut-brain axis is particularly sensitive to stress. Stress signals from the brain can affect gut function, leading to symptoms such as bloating, stomach cramps, or changes in bowel habits. Conversely, a distressed gut can send signals to the brain, influencing mood and stress responses.

5. Immune System Crosstalk:

The gut and the brain are intertwined with the immune system, with immune cells patrolling both the gastrointestinal tract and the central nervous system. Dysregulation in the gut can trigger an immune response that may impact the brain, contributing to inflammation and potential neurological consequences.

6. Dietary Impact:

The foods we consume play a pivotal role in shaping the gut microbiota and, consequently, the gut-brain connection. Diets rich in fiber, prebiotics, and probiotics support a diverse and healthy microbiota, fostering positive interactions with the brain.

7. Implications for Mental Health Interventions:

The growing understanding of the gut-brain connection opens new avenues for mental health interventions. Probiotics, prebiotics, and dietary strategies that promote a healthy gut microbiota are areas of exploration for researchers seeking novel approaches to support mental well-being.

8. Lifestyle Factors:

Lifestyle factors, including sleep, exercise, and stress management, also influence the gut-brain connection. Prioritizing a holistic approach to health that encompasses these factors contributes to the overall balance of the gut-brain axis.

In conclusion, the gut-brain connection serves as a testament to the interconnectedness of bodily systems. It is becoming more and more clear how important it is to support both gastrointestinal and mental health as research into this complex link evolves. Recognizing the profound impact of lifestyle, diet, and stress management on the gut-brain axis empowers individuals to take proactive steps in fostering not just physical health but also the resilience and vitality of the mind. Discovering a harmonious gut-brain connection is an intriguing journey at the junction of neuroscience, biology, and holistic health.

Nutrients and Cognitive Function

Nutrients and Cognitive Function: Fueling the Mind for Optimal Performance

The complex interplay between nutrition and cognitive function highlights the significant influence of dietary choices on mental clarity, memory, and general brain health. As the command center of the body, the brain requires a diverse array of nutrients to function optimally, emphasizing the critical role of nutrition in sustaining cognitive abilities throughout life.

1. Omega-3 Fatty Acids:

Essential Brain Boosters: Omega-3 fatty acids, particularly docosahexaenoic acid (DHA) and eicosapentaenoic acid (EPA), are fundamental components of brain cell membranes. Found in fatty fish, walnuts, and flaxseeds, these fatty acids play a crucial role in supporting cognitive functions, including memory and problem-solving skills.

2. Antioxidants:

Guardians Against Oxidative Stress: Antioxidants, abundant in fruits and vegetables, act as defenders against oxidative stress—a process linked to cognitive decline and neurodegenerative diseases. Vitamins C and E, as well as compounds like flavonoids, contribute to a protective shield for the brain.

3. B Vitamins:

Metabolic Enablers: B vitamins, including B6, B9 (folate), and B12, are vital for brain health. They play key roles in neurotransmitter synthesis and help regulate homocysteine levels, an amino acid associated with cognitive decline. Leafy greens, legumes, and lean meats are rich sources.

4. Vitamin D:

Sunshine Vitamin for Cognitive Health: Vitamin D, often associated with bone health, also plays a role in cognitive function. Adequate levels of vitamin D, obtained from sunlight exposure and dietary sources like fatty fish and fortified dairy products, are linked to better cognitive performance.

5. Iron:

Oxygen Transport for Brain Vitality: Iron is essential for oxygen transport to the brain. A deficiency can lead to cognitive impairment and fatigue. Red meat, poultry, beans, and fortified cereals are excellent sources of iron, supporting cognitive vitality.

6. Zinc:

Crucial for Memory and Learning: Zinc is involved in neurotransmitter function and has a pivotal role in memory and learning. Foods such as meat, dairy, nuts, and legumes provide the necessary zinc for optimal cognitive function.

7. Magnesium:

Neurotransmitter Regulation: Magnesium plays a role in regulating neurotransmitters and supporting synaptic plasticity—the ability of brain synapses to strengthen or weaken over time. Leafy greens, nuts, and whole grains are magnesium-rich foods.

8. Protein:

Amino Acids for Neurotransmitters: Proteins provide the amino acids required for neurotransmitter synthesis. Including lean meats, dairy, eggs, and plant-based protein sources ensures a balanced intake to support cognitive functions.

9. Hydration:

Fluids for Cognitive Clarity: Dehydration can impair cognitive function, affecting concentration and memory. Staying well-hydrated by consuming water and other hydrating beverages supports optimal brain function.

10. Polyphenols:

Brain-Boosting Plant Compounds: Polyphenols found in tea, coffee, berries, and dark chocolate exhibit neuroprotective properties. They may contribute to improved cognitive performance and potentially reduce the risk of neurodegenerative diseases.

The relationship between nutrients and cognitive function is a dynamic and multifaceted alliance that underscores the importance of a well-balanced and varied diet. By incorporating nutrient-rich foods into our daily meals, we not only nourish our bodies but also fortify the cognitive machinery that propels us through the intricate landscape of thought, memory, and learning.

Nutrition and Mood Disorders

Nourishing the Mind: The Role of Nutrition in Managing Mood Disorders

The relationship between nutrition and mental health should be studied in-depth when addressing mood disorders. While medical interventions and therapeutic approaches play crucial roles, the impact of dietary choices on mood regulation and emotional well-being cannot be overlooked. In this section, we delve into the connection between nutrition and mood disorders, emphasizing the role of a balanced and mindful diet in supporting mental health.

1. Omega-3 Fatty Acids:

Brain-Boosting Lipids: Omega-3 fatty acids, found abundantly in fatty fish, flaxseeds, and walnuts, have been associated with reduced symptoms of depression and anxiety. These essential fats contribute to the structural integrity of brain cells and play a role in neurotransmitter function.

2. Complex Carbohydrates:

Steady Energy, Stable Mood: Incorporating complex carbohydrates, such as whole grains, legumes, and vegetables, into the diet helps regulate blood sugar levels. This steady release of energy can prevent mood swings and support a more stable emotional state.

3. Lean Proteins:

Amino Acids for Neurotransmitters: Protein-rich foods provide essential amino acids necessary for neurotransmitter synthesis. Lean meats, poultry, fish, eggs, and plant-based protein sources contribute to a balanced mood by supporting neurotransmitter balance.

4. Serotonin-Boosting Foods:

The Serotonin Connection: Foods rich in tryptophan, a precursor to serotonin, can positively influence mood. Turkey, chicken, dairy products, nuts, and seeds are examples of tryptophan-containing foods that contribute to serotonin production.

5. Fruits and Vegetables:

Antioxidants for Emotional Resilience: The vibrant colors of fruits and vegetables indicate the presence of antioxidants, which combat oxidative stress. Antioxidants have been linked to improved mood and a reduced risk of mood disorders.

6. B Vitamins:

Mood-Regulating Nutrients: B vitamins, particularly B6, B9 (folate), and B12, play essential roles in neurotransmitter synthesis. Deficiencies in these vitamins have been associated with an increased risk of mood disorders, making foods like leafy greens, legumes, and fortified cereals important for mental well-being.

7. Probiotics and Gut Health:

The Gut-Brain Axis: Emerging research suggests a link between gut health and mood regulation. Probiotics, found in fermented foods like yogurt and kimchi, promote a healthy gut microbiome, potentially influencing mood and emotional resilience.

8. Hydration:

Water for Mental Clarity: Dehydration can negatively impact mood and cognitive function. Staying well-hydrated by consuming water throughout the day is a simple yet effective way to support mental well-being.

9. Limiting Sugar and Processed Foods:

The Impact of Processed Foods: Excessive consumption of sugary and processed foods has been linked to an increased risk of mood disorders. A diet rich in whole, unprocessed foods provides a more stable foundation for emotional balance.

10. Mindful Eating Practices:

Connection Between Body and Mind: Engaging in mindful eating practices, such as savoring each bite and being attuned to hunger and fullness cues, fosters a positive relationship with food. This mindful approach to eating can contribute to emotional well-being.

In conclusion, while nutrition cannot replace professional medical care for mood disorders, it serves as a crucial adjunct in managing symptoms and supporting overall mental health. A well-rounded, nutrient-dense diet provides the foundation for emotional resilience and mood regulation. As individuals navigate the complexities of mood disorders, incorporating these nutritional principles into their lifestyle can become a powerful ally in their journey toward mental well-being. Always consult healthcare professionals for personalized guidance and treatment plans tailored to your body's specific needs.

Chapter 11

Specialized Diets

Specialized diets encompass tailored nutritional approaches designed to address specific health goals, dietary preferences, or medical conditions. One such example is the ketogenic diet, characterized by high fat and low carbohydrate intake, promoting a state of ketosis for energy production. Often associated with weight loss and improved blood sugar control, the keto diet demands meticulous planning to avoid nutrient deficiencies and potential adaptation challenges.

Another noteworthy specialized diet is the paleo diet, inspired by the dietary patterns of our ancestors. It emphasizes whole foods like lean meats, fruits, and vegetables, aiming to reduce inflammation and promote nutrient-dense eating. While lauded for its potential benefits, considerations include the risk of protein overload and the need for adaptation to individual preferences.

The Mediterranean diet, rooted in the traditional eating habits of Mediterranean countries, features fruits, vegetables, whole grains, fish, and olive oil. Recognized for its heart health advantages, this diet underscores the importance of balance and moderation. However, interpretations may vary, and individuals with specific dietary restrictions must exercise caution.

Specialized diets extend to plant-based lifestyles, such as the vegan diet, which excludes all animal products. Though associated with sustainability and reduced disease risk, meticulous planning is crucial to addressing potential nutrient deficiencies.

Gluten-Free

A gluten-free diet involves the exclusion of gluten, a protein found in wheat, barley, rye, and their derivatives. This dietary approach is essential for individuals with celiac disease, a genetic autoimmune condition in which the ingestion of gluten triggers an immune response that damages the small intestine. For these individuals, adhering to a strict gluten-free diet is the only effective treatment.

Importance of a Gluten-Free Diet:

Celiac Disease Management: The primary medical indication for a gluten-free diet is to manage celiac disease. Consumption of gluten by individuals with celiac disease can lead to severe intestinal damage, malabsorption of nutrients, and various health complications.

Symptom Relief: Beyond celiac disease, some individuals may have non-celiac gluten sensitivity, experiencing gastrointestinal or extra-intestinal symptoms when gluten is consumed. A gluten-free diet can alleviate these symptoms.

Dermatitis Herpetiformis Treatment: Dermatitis Herpetiformis is a skin condition associated with celiac disease. A gluten-free diet is crucial in managing and preventing the skin lesions characteristic of this condition.

Wheat Allergy Management: In cases of wheat allergy, which is different from gluten intolerance or celiac disease, a gluten-free diet may be recommended to eliminate the source of the allergic reaction.

Autoimmune Disorders: Some autoimmune conditions, such as rheumatoid arthritis or lupus, may benefit from a gluten-free diet, although the evidence is not conclusive. Some individuals report symptom improvement, but more research is needed in this area.

It's important to note that a gluten-free diet can be challenging to maintain, as gluten is present in many commonly consumed foods. Individuals considering this diet should seek guidance from healthcare professionals or registered dietitians to ensure nutritional adequacy and proper management of their specific health conditions. For those without gluten-related disorders, adopting a gluten-free diet may not offer additional health benefits and could potentially lead to nutritional imbalances.

Veganism and Vegetarianism

Vegetarianism:

Vegetarianism is a dietary practice that abstains from the consumption of meat, poultry, and seafood. Vegetarians primarily rely on plant-based foods, including fruits, vegetables, grains, legumes, nuts, and seeds. There are various forms of vegetarianism, with some individuals including dairy products and eggs in their diet (lacto-ovo vegetarians), while others exclude one or both of these categories (vegans). The decision to follow a vegetarian diet is often influenced by ethical, environmental, health, or cultural considerations.

Veganism:

Veganism is a more restrictive dietary and lifestyle choice that eliminates all animal-derived products. In addition to avoiding meat, poultry, and seafood, vegans exclude dairy, eggs, honey, and other animal by-products. Veganism extends beyond diet to embrace a philosophy that seeks to minimize harm to animals in all aspects of life, including clothing, cosmetics, and household products. Vegans rely solely on plant-based sources for their nutritional needs, emphasizing fruits, vegetables, grains, legumes, nuts, and seeds.

The trend of veganism has gained significant traction in recent years, driven by a combination of ethical, environmental, and health considerations. Several factors contribute to the increasing popularity of veganism, including:

1. Ethical and Animal Welfare Concerns:

A growing awareness of factory farming practices and the treatment of animals has led many individuals to adopt veganism as a stance against animal cruelty. Documentaries and social media have played a role in exposing the conditions in which animals are often raised for food production, influencing people to seek alternatives.

2. Environmental Sustainability:

The environmental impact of animal agriculture, including deforestation, water consumption, and greenhouse gas emissions, has become a prominent concern. As people become more environmentally conscious, choosing a vegan lifestyle is seen as a way to reduce one's ecological footprint and promote sustainability.

3. Health and Wellness Trends:

The association between plant-based diets and various health benefits, including lower risks of heart disease, diabetes, and certain cancers, has contributed to the popularity of veganism. Many individuals are adopting a vegan lifestyle as part of a broader focus on health and wellness.

4. Celebrity Influence:

Influential celebrities and public figures adopting veganism have brought the lifestyle into the mainstream spotlight. Their endorsement and promotion of plant-based diets through social media and other platforms contribute to the trend's visibility and acceptance.

5. Availability of Plant-Based Alternatives:

The increased availability and accessibility of plant-based alternatives to traditional animal products have made it easier for individuals to transition to a vegan lifestyle. Plant-based options in supermarkets, restaurants, and cafes are expanding, catering to the growing demand.

6. Social Media and Information Sharing:

Social media platforms serve as powerful tools for information sharing and community building. Vegan influencers and activists use these platforms to share recipes, tips, and information about the benefits of veganism, creating a sense of community and encouraging more people to join the movement.

7. Documentary Impact:

Documentaries such as "Cowspiracy," "Forks Over Knives," and "What the Health" have shed light on the environmental, ethical, and health implications of animal agriculture. These documentaries have sparked conversations and prompted individuals to reconsider their dietary choices.

8. Corporate and Restaurant Adoption:

Major corporations and restaurant chains incorporating vegan options into their menus reflect the mainstream acceptance of plant-based diets. The presence of vegan choices in popular food establishments makes it more convenient for people to embrace veganism.

The combination of ethical considerations, environmental awareness, health consciousness, and increased accessibility to plant-based alternatives has propelled veganism into a prominent and influential trend that continues to shape dietary choices and lifestyles globally.

Both vegetarianism and veganism have gained popularity for their potential health benefits, ethical considerations related to animal welfare, and environmental sustainability. Individuals often choose these dietary paths based on personal beliefs, health objectives, and concerns about the environmental impact of animal agriculture. It's essential for those adopting these diets to plan their nutrition carefully to ensure the intake of all essential nutrients. Consulting with healthcare professionals or registered dietitians can provide guidance on achieving a balanced and healthy plant-based diet.

Ketogenic Diet

The ketogenic diet, often referred to as the keto diet, is a high-fat, low-carbohydrate diet designed to induce a metabolic state known as ketosis. In ketosis, the body shifts its primary source of energy from glucose (derived from carbohydrates) to ketones (produced from fats). This shift prompts the body to burn stored fat for fuel, leading to weight loss and other potential health benefits.

Key Components of the Ketogenic Diet:

High Fat: The diet typically consists of approximately 70-80% of calories from fats, including sources like avocados, nuts, seeds, and oils.

Low Carbohydrate: Carbohydrate intake is restricted to around 5-10% of total calories. This limitation aims to deplete glycogen stores, encouraging the body to use fats for energy.

Moderate Protein: Protein intake is moderate, comprising about 20-25% of total calories. It is essential for maintaining muscle mass and overall body function.

Significance of the Ketogenic Diet:

Weight Loss: One of the primary reasons people adopt the ketogenic diet is for weight loss. The shift to fat metabolism can lead to a reduction in body fat, especially in individuals with obesity.

Blood Sugar Control: The ketogenic diet may help stabilize blood sugar levels and improve insulin sensitivity, making it potentially beneficial for individuals with type 2 diabetes or those at risk of developing the condition.

Increased Satiety: The high-fat content of the diet, combined with the production of ketones, may contribute to increased feelings of fullness and reduced appetite, aiding in weight management.

Enhanced Mental Clarity: Some individuals on the ketogenic diet report improved mental clarity and focus. The brain can efficiently utilize ketones as an alternative energy source.

Epilepsy Treatment: The ketogenic diet has been used as a therapeutic approach for epilepsy, especially in children. It can help reduce the frequency and severity of seizures in some cases.

Potential Cardiovascular Benefits: While controversial, some studies suggest that the ketogenic diet may positively impact cardiovascular risk factors, such as improving lipid profiles and reducing inflammation.

Neurological Conditions: Research is ongoing to explore the potential benefits of the ketogenic diet for various neurological conditions, including Alzheimer's disease and Parkinson's disease.

It's important to note that the ketogenic diet is not suitable for everyone, and its long-term effects and potential risks are areas of ongoing research. Individuals considering this diet should consult with healthcare professionals or registered dietitians to ensure it aligns with their health goals and is implemented safely and effectively.

Intermittent Fasting

Intermittent fasting (IF) is an eating pattern that cycles between periods of eating and fasting. Unlike traditional diets that focus on what to eat, intermittent fasting emphasizes when to eat. It doesn't prescribe specific foods but rather designates specific windows for eating and fasting. There are several methods of intermittent fasting, and individuals can choose the one that fits their lifestyle and preferences.

Common Methods of Intermittent Fasting:

16/8 Method: Involves daily fasting for 16 hours and restricting eating to an 8-hour window. For example, eating between 12:00 pm and 8:00 pm and fasting from 8:00 pm to 12:00 pm the next day.

5:2 Diet: Involves consuming a regular diet for five days of the week and drastically reducing calorie intake (around 500-600 calories) on the other two non-consecutive days.

Eat-Stop-Eat: Requires a 24-hour fast once or twice a week. For instance, fasting from dinner one day to dinner the next day.

Alternate-Day Fasting: Involves alternating between days of regular eating and days of either very low-calorie intake or complete fasting.

Significance of Intermittent Fasting:

Weight Loss: Intermittent fasting can be an effective strategy for weight loss by reducing overall calorie intake and promoting fat loss. During fasting periods, the body utilizes stored energy, contributing to weight loss.

Improved Insulin Sensitivity: IF may enhance insulin sensitivity, potentially lowering the risk of type 2 diabetes. Fasting periods help regulate blood sugar levels and reduce insulin resistance.

Cellular Repair and Autophagy: Fasting triggers a process called autophagy, where cells remove damaged components and regenerate. This cellular repair mechanism is associated with longevity and a reduced risk of various diseases.

Heart Health: IF may have cardiovascular benefits by improving lipid profiles, reducing inflammation, and supporting heart health. It may contribute to lowering risk factors for heart disease.

Brain Health: Some studies suggest that intermittent fasting may have neuroprotective effects, promoting brain health and potentially reducing the risk of neurodegenerative diseases.

Simplicity and Flexibility: Intermittent fasting is relatively simple to implement, requiring no specific meal planning or calorie counting. It offers flexibility in choosing the fasting method that suits individual preferences and schedules.

Hormonal Benefits: IF may positively influence hormonal balance, including increased levels of norepinephrine and human growth hormone, which play roles in metabolism and fat burning.

Longevity: While research on humans is ongoing, some animal studies suggest that intermittent fasting may contribute to an increased lifespan and a reduction in age-related diseases.

It's essential to note that intermittent fasting may not be suitable for everyone, and individual responses can vary. Before starting any fasting regimen, it's advisable to consult with healthcare professionals, especially for individuals with underlying health conditions or specific dietary needs.

Chapter 12

Nutrition and Weight Management

The Crucial Role of Nutrition in Effective Weight Management

Achieving and maintaining a healthy weight is a complex journey that involves a combination of factors, with nutrition playing a pivotal role. Proper nutrition not only supports overall well-being but is also instrumental in effective weight management. This section explores the relationship between nutrition and weight, highlighting key principles and strategies to promote a balanced and sustainable approach to achieving and maintaining a healthy body weight.

The Basics of Nutrition:

Caloric Balance: Weight management is fundamentally linked to the balance between calories consumed and calories expended. Consuming more calories than the body needs leads to weight gain, while a calorie deficit results in weight loss. Establishing a healthy balance is essential.

Macronutrients: Understanding and incorporating the right mix of macronutrients—carbohydrates, proteins, and fats—is crucial. Each plays a unique role in metabolism, energy production, and satiety. Striking a balance based on individual needs and goals is key.

Micronutrients: Essential vitamins and minerals are vital for overall health. They contribute to metabolic processes, immune function, and various physiological functions. A well-rounded, nutrient-dense diet ensures the body receives the necessary micronutrients for optimal functioning.

Nutrition and Weight Loss:

Mindful Eating: Developing awareness of hunger and satiety cues promotes mindful eating. Paying attention to portion sizes and savoring each bite can prevent overeating and foster a healthier relationship with food.

Balanced Diets: Fad diets often promise quick fixes, but they are rarely sustainable. Instead, focus on balanced diets that include a variety of foods, emphasizing fruits, vegetables, whole grains, lean proteins, and healthy fats.

Hydration: Adequate water intake is often overlooked but is essential for weight management. Water supports metabolism, helps control hunger, and aids in digestion. Opting for water over sugary beverages can significantly impact caloric intake.

Nutrition and Weight Maintenance:

Lifestyle Habits: Sustainable weight management involves adopting healthy lifestyle habits. Regular physical activity, sufficient sleep, and stress management contribute to overall well-being and help maintain a healthy weight.

Long-Term Perspective: Weight management is a journey, not a destination. Embrace a long-term perspective, focusing on gradual, sustainable changes. Small, consistent adjustments in eating habits and physical activity yield lasting results.

Professional Guidance: Seek professional guidance from a registered dietician or a nutritionist to get a diet plan that's customized to your needs based on several other factors, including your BMI, metabolism, age, gender, and health issues, etc.

Adopting a balanced, mindful approach to eating, coupled with lifestyle habits that support overall health, paves the way for sustainable weight loss and maintenance. Remember, the goal is not just to shed pounds temporarily but to cultivate habits that promote a lifetime of health and well-being.

Healthy Approaches to Weight Loss

Embarking on a weight loss journey is a common goal for many individuals seeking to enhance their overall health. However, the path to shedding excess pounds should prioritize sustainable and healthy approaches over quick fixes. This article explores effective and balanced strategies for achieving weight loss while prioritizing well-being and long-term success.

Set Realistic Goals: Establishing realistic and achievable weight loss goals is paramount. Rather than aiming for rapid results, focus on gradual, steady progress. Sustainable weight loss typically ranges from 0.5 to 2 pounds per week.

Mindful Eating: Cultivate mindfulness around eating habits. Pay attention to hunger and fullness cues, savor each bite, and avoid distractions during meals. This approach encourages a healthier relationship with food and can prevent overeating.

Balanced Nutrition: Adopt a balanced and varied diet that includes a mix of fruits, vegetables, whole grains, lean proteins, and healthy fats. Prioritize nutrient-dense foods to ensure the body receives essential vitamins and minerals while managing caloric intake.

Portion Control: Be mindful of portion sizes to avoid overconsumption. Use smaller plates, pay attention to serving sizes, and resist the urge to go back for seconds immediately. Portion control is a key component of sustainable weight management.

Regular Physical Activity: Incorporate regular physical activity into your routine. Aim for a combination of aerobic exercises, strength training, and flexibility exercises. Find activities you enjoy to make exercise a sustainable and enjoyable part of your lifestyle.

Stay Hydrated: Drinking an adequate amount of water supports weight loss by promoting satiety and boosting metabolism. Replace sugary beverages with water to reduce unnecessary calorie intake.

Sleep Quality: Prioritize sufficient and quality sleep. Lack of sleep can disrupt hormonal balance, leading to increased appetite and cravings. Aim for 7-9 hours of sleep per night to support overall well-being and weight loss efforts.

Stress Management:

Chronic stress can contribute to weight gain. Incorporate stress-reducing practices such as meditation, deep breathing exercises, or yoga into your routine. Managing stress is crucial for both mental and physical health.

Social Support:

Share your weight loss journey with friends or family for added accountability and support. Surrounding yourself with a positive and encouraging social network can make the process more enjoyable and sustainable.

Seek Professional Guidance:

Consult with healthcare professionals, registered dietitians, or certified fitness trainers for personalized advice. They can help tailor a plan based on your individual needs, taking into account factors such as medical history and lifestyle.

Healthy weight loss is not just about shedding pounds; it's about adopting a sustainable and balanced lifestyle that promotes overall well-being. By incorporating mindful eating, regular physical activity, and other health-focused strategies, individuals can achieve their weight loss goals in a manner that enhances rather than compromises their health. Remember, the journey to a healthier you is a marathon, not a sprint.

Breaking Myths about Fad Diets

In a world where quick fixes and instant results are often sought after, fad diets have gained popularity. However, behind the promises of rapid weight loss, these diets often harbor myths and misconceptions. This article aims to shed light on some of the most common myths surrounding fad diets, emphasizing the importance of evidence-based approaches to nutrition and weight management.

Myth: Fad Diets Guarantee Quick and Sustainable Weight Loss:

Fact: While fad diets may lead to initial weight loss, they often lack sustainability. Many of these diets are restrictive and eliminate entire food groups, making it challenging to maintain over the long term. Sustainable weight loss requires a balanced and realistic approach.

Myth: Cutting Out Entire Food Groups is Healthy:

Fact: Fad diets often advocate for eliminating entire food groups, such as carbohydrates or fats. However, each food group plays a crucial role in providing essential nutrients. A balanced diet that includes a variety of foods ensures the body receives the necessary vitamins, minerals, and macronutrients.

Myth: Fad Diets Detoxify the Body:

Fact: The concept of detoxifying the body through extreme diets or juice cleanses lacks scientific support. The human body has its own built-in detoxification systems, primarily the liver and kidneys, which work continuously to eliminate toxins. A well-balanced diet supports these natural processes.

Myth: One Size Fits All:

Fact: Fad diets often claim to be universally effective, overlooking individual differences in metabolism, genetics, and lifestyle. What works for one person may not work for another. Personalized and evidence-based approaches are essential for sustainable results.

Myth: Fad Diets Are the Only Solution for Weight Loss:

Fact: There is no one-size-fits-all solution for weight loss. Sustainable and effective weight management involves adopting a holistic approach that includes balanced nutrition, regular physical activity, and healthy lifestyle habits. Fad diets are not the only, nor the healthiest, path to weight loss.

Myth: Skipping Meals Speeds Up Weight Loss:

Fact: Skipping meals can lead to nutrient deficiencies and disrupt metabolism. While it may result in a short-term calorie reduction, it often leads to overeating later in the day. Eating regular, balanced meals supports sustainable weight loss by maintaining energy levels and preventing excessive hunger.

Myth: Fad Diets Provide Long-Term Health Benefits:

Fact: Fad diets may lead to temporary weight loss, but they often lack the nutrients needed for long-term health. Some extreme diets can even contribute to nutrient deficiencies, negatively impacting overall well-being. A focus on balanced nutrition and lifestyle changes is crucial for lasting health benefits.

Breaking free from the myths surrounding fad diets is essential for making informed choices about weight management and overall health. Embracing evidence-based, sustainable approaches that prioritize balanced nutrition, regular physical activity, and a healthy lifestyle leads to long-lasting well-being without falling prey to the allure of quick fixes. Remember, the key to a healthy and fulfilling life lies in adopting habits that can be maintained for the long haul.

Building a Sustainable and Balanced Lifestyle

The pursuit of a healthy, sustainable lifestyle is more important than ever in the hustle and bustle of our hectic lives. Constructing a foundation that harmonizes physical, mental, and emotional well-being is not only desirable but essential for a fulfilling life. At the core of this endeavor lies the commitment to regular physical activity, a cornerstone of a healthy lifestyle. Incorporating a mix of aerobic exercises, strength training, and flexibility routines not only enhances physical health but also contributes to mental clarity and emotional resilience.

Complementing a physically active routine is a crucial element of balanced nutrition. A well-rounded, nutrient-dense diet rich in fruits, vegetables, whole grains, lean proteins, and healthy fats provides the body with the fuel it needs for optimal functioning. Striving for moderation rather than strict restrictions allows for a sustainable approach to eating, fostering a positive relationship with food. Equally important is the recognition of the vital role sleep plays in our overall well-being. Prioritizing quality sleep through consistent sleep schedules and creating a sleep-friendly environment supports cognitive function, emotional stability, and physical recovery.

Stress management becomes a linchpin in the pursuit of balance. Integrating stress-reducing practices such as meditation, deep breathing exercises, or yoga into our daily lives fosters emotional resilience and mental well-being. Mindful eating practices, emphasizing present-moment awareness during meals, not only enhance our connection with food but also prevent overeating by attuning us to hunger and fullness cues. Hydration, often underestimated, is another key element. Maintaining adequate water intake supports bodily functions, aids digestion, and ensures sustained energy levels.

Beyond the individual components of a healthy lifestyle, the cultivation of meaningful relationships plays a pivotal role. Nurturing connections with family, friends, and community fosters emotional well-being and provides a support system during life's challenges. Embracing a continuous learning mindset, whether through pursuing new hobbies, reading, or taking courses, contributes to intellectual stimulation and personal growth. Establishing clear boundaries between work and personal life promotes a healthy work-life balance, allowing time for relaxation, leisure, and personal pursuits.

Ultimately, the journey toward building a sustainable, balanced lifestyle involves setting realistic goals aligned with one's values. Breaking down larger aspirations into smaller, achievable steps allows for steady progress, accompanied by a sense of accomplishment and motivation. In this ongoing process, the key is to find a balance that resonates with individual needs and aspirations, creating a framework for a fulfilling and healthy life. As we navigate the complexities of modern living, our commitment to these principles becomes a compass, guiding us toward a lifestyle that stands the test of time.

Chapter 13

Global Nutrition Challenges

In an interconnected world facing rapid demographic, economic, and environmental changes, global nutrition challenges have emerged as significant obstacles to public health. Addressing these challenges requires collaborative efforts, innovative solutions, and a collective commitment to fostering sustainable nutritional practices.

Malnutrition in All its Forms:

Malnutrition extends beyond the stereotypical image of undernourished individuals; it encapsulates both undernutrition and overnutrition. While millions suffer from hunger and a lack of essential nutrients, a parallel challenge arises with the increasing prevalence of obesity and diet-related non-communicable diseases. Tackling malnutrition in all its forms demands a holistic approach that addresses food security, nutritional education, and access to diverse and nutritious diets.

Food Insecurity and Unequal Access:

The global challenge of food insecurity persists, affecting millions who lack consistent access to sufficient, safe, and nutritious food. Disparities in food access exist both within and among nations, exacerbating social inequalities. Initiatives that promote sustainable agriculture, equitable distribution systems, and community-based interventions are essential to alleviate this pressing issue.

Micronutrient Deficiencies:

Micronutrient deficiencies, often referred to as "hidden hunger," remain prevalent worldwide. Inadequate intake of essential vitamins and minerals contributes to a range of health issues, affecting vulnerable populations, particularly children and pregnant women. Promoting diversified diets, fortifying staple foods, and public health campaigns can help combat micronutrient deficiencies.

Rising Impact of Climate Change:

Climate change poses a growing threat to global nutrition. Extreme weather events, shifting agricultural patterns, and environmental degradation compromise the availability and nutritional quality of food. A comprehensive response involves sustainable agricultural practices, resilient food systems, and efforts to mitigate the impact of climate change on nutrition.

Unhealthy Diets and Lifestyle Diseases:

The globalization of unhealthy dietary patterns, characterized by the increased consumption of processed foods, sugary beverages, and high-calorie diets, contributes to a rise in non-communicable diseases such as diabetes and cardiovascular issues. Shifting societal norms toward healthier eating habits, alongside policies that regulate food marketing and labeling, is crucial for preventing diet-related diseases.

Limited Access to Clean Water and Sanitation:

Access to clean water and sanitation is foundational to good nutrition and health. Millions lack these basic necessities, leading to waterborne diseases and hindering proper hygiene practices. Comprehensive strategies must integrate nutrition and water sanitation interventions to ensure holistic well-being.

Addressing global nutrition challenges requires a multifaceted and collaborative approach that encompasses policy changes, community engagement, and international cooperation. As we confront the complexities of malnutrition, unequal food access, micronutrient deficiencies, climate change impacts, unhealthy dietary trends, and limited access to clean water, it is crucial to recognize the interconnected nature of these issues. A commitment to sustainable solutions, informed by evidence-based practices, can pave the way for a healthier, more equitable global society. In this shared journey toward improved nutrition, individuals, communities, governments, and international organizations all play vital roles in shaping a brighter, healthier future for all.

Malnutrition and Hunger

In a world abundant with resources, the persistent challenges of malnutrition and hunger cast a shadow over the well-being of millions. Malnutrition, a complex issue, encompasses both undernutrition and overnutrition, affecting diverse populations across the globe.

Undernutrition: A Silent Crisis:

At the heart of malnutrition lies the silent crisis of undernutrition. Millions, particularly in developing regions, face insufficient intake of essential nutrients, leading to stunted growth, compromised immune systems, and developmental delays. Insufficient access to diverse and nutritious foods, compounded by factors such as poverty and a lack of education, contributes to this pervasive challenge.

Overnutrition and the Rise of Obesity:

Simultaneously, the world witnesses the alarming rise of overnutrition, where individuals consume an excess of calories, often derived from unhealthy, processed foods. This contributes to the global obesity epidemic, fostering a range of non-communicable diseases such as diabetes, cardiovascular issues, and certain cancers. The coexistence of undernutrition and overnutrition within communities highlights the complex and interconnected nature of malnutrition.

Food Insecurity: A Barrier to Well-Being:

Hunger, a poignant consequence of malnutrition, persists as a global challenge. Food insecurity, characterized by inadequate access to sufficient, safe, and nutritious food, plagues communities worldwide. Vulnerable populations, including children, pregnant women, and the elderly, face the harsh reality of going without a reliable source of nourishment, impacting not only their physical health but also their educational and economic prospects.

Impact on Child Development:

Malnutrition, particularly during the critical early years of life, can have lasting consequences on a child's development. Stunted growth, cognitive impairments, and increased vulnerability to diseases impede a child's ability to thrive and reach their full potential. Breaking the cycle of malnutrition requires a holistic approach that addresses not only immediate nutritional needs but also underlying socio-economic factors.

Global Efforts and Sustainable Solutions:

Tackling malnutrition and hunger demands a collective commitment from governments, NGOs, the private sector, and individuals. International initiatives, such as the Sustainable Development Goals, highlight the importance of eradicating hunger, achieving food security, improving nutrition, and promoting sustainable agriculture. Policies that address social inequalities, promote education, and ensure access to healthcare are integral components of sustainable solutions.

Community Empowerment and Education:

At the grassroots level, community empowerment and education play pivotal roles in combating malnutrition. Programs that educate communities about balanced nutrition, sustainable farming practices, and efficient food distribution empower individuals to take control of their nutritional well-being. By fostering self-sufficiency and resilience, communities can break free from the cycle of hunger and malnutrition.

Malnutrition and hunger are challenges that transcend borders and demand a united, global response. By understanding the complex interplay of factors contributing to undernutrition and overnutrition, we can pave the way for comprehensive solutions that address immediate needs while promoting long-term sustainability. As a global community, we must strive toward a future where no one suffers the debilitating effects of hunger, and every individual has the opportunity to lead a healthy, productive life. By working together, educating people, and being devoted to social justice, we can change the story and make food insecurity a thing of the past.

Obesity Epidemic

In recent decades, the global prevalence of obesity has surged, presenting a complex and pervasive health challenge that extends across borders, affecting individuals of all ages, ethnicities, and socio-economic backgrounds. This article delves into the multifaceted nature of the obesity epidemic, exploring its causes, consequences, and the imperative need for collective efforts to address and reverse this global health crisis.

Rising Prevalence and Health Impacts:

The obesity epidemic has reached alarming proportions, with a significant increase in the number of individuals classified as overweight or obese. Beyond its societal implications, obesity takes a toll on individual health, increasing the risk of chronic conditions such as diabetes, cardiovascular diseases, certain cancers, and musculoskeletal disorders.

Root Causes:

The complex etiology of obesity involves a combination of genetic, environmental, and behavioral factors. Sedentary lifestyles, high-calorie diets rich in processed foods, and increased screen time contribute to an imbalance between calorie intake and expenditure. Socio-economic factors, such as limited access to healthy foods and opportunities for physical activity, further exacerbate the issue.

Childhood Obesity: A Growing Concern:

The prevalence of obesity among children and adolescents is of particular concern. Early-onset obesity not only increases the risk of immediate health issues but also sets the stage for a lifelong struggle with weight management. Addressing childhood obesity is crucial for breaking the cycle and promoting long-term health.

Societal and Environmental Influences:

Societal factors, including urbanization, marketing of unhealthy foods, and built environments that discourage physical activity, play a significant role in the obesity epidemic. Efforts to create healthier communities must involve policy changes, such as improved urban planning, regulation of food marketing, and the creation of safe spaces for physical activity.

Psychosocial Aspects:

Obesity is not solely a physical health concern; it also carries psychosocial implications. Individuals facing obesity may encounter stigmatization, discrimination, and challenges in accessing healthcare. Addressing the psychosocial aspects of obesity requires fostering a culture of empathy, inclusivity, and understanding.

Global Economic Burden:

The economic impact of the obesity epidemic is substantial, affecting healthcare systems, productivity, and overall economic well-being. The costs associated with treating obesity-related diseases and the loss of productivity due to health issues contribute to a significant economic burden on societies worldwide.

Prevention and Intervention Strategies:

Combating the obesity epidemic necessitates a comprehensive approach that spans prevention and intervention strategies. Promoting healthier eating habits, increasing physical activity opportunities, and creating environments conducive to a balanced lifestyle are pivotal. Additionally, early intervention, personalized healthcare approaches, and community-based initiatives are essential components of a multifaceted solution.

Addressing the obesity epidemic requires a collective, multidisciplinary effort that extends beyond individual choices to encompass societal, environmental, and policy-level changes. By fostering awareness, implementing evidence-based interventions, and promoting a culture of health, we can work towards reversing the obesity epidemic and ensuring a healthier future for generations to come. Through shared responsibility, education, and a commitment to wellness, we can transform the narrative surrounding obesity and build a world where health is prioritized, and individuals are empowered to lead fulfilling lives.

Addressing Global Food Insecurity

In a world capable of producing an abundance of food, the persistent challenge of global food insecurity remains a stark reality. Millions of people worldwide face insufficient access to safe, nutritious, and affordable food, posing profound threats to health, development, and social equity. Let's explore the multifaceted issue of global food insecurity, delving into its root causes, consequences, and the imperative need for concerted, sustainable efforts to ensure that no one goes hungry.

Understanding Food Insecurity:

Food insecurity goes beyond a mere lack of food; it encompasses a spectrum of challenges ranging from insufficient quantity and quality of food to uncertainties about its availability. Affected individuals and communities often grapple with the uncertainty of securing their next meal, leading to malnutrition, stunted growth, and compromised overall well-being.

Root Causes:

A myriad of interconnected factors contributes to global food insecurity. Poverty, conflict, climate change, inadequate infrastructure, and the uneven distribution of resources are key drivers. In regions experiencing armed conflicts or climate-related disasters, access to food becomes even more precarious, exacerbating existing vulnerabilities.

Impact on Vulnerable Populations:

Vulnerable populations, including children, pregnant women, and the elderly, are disproportionately affected by food insecurity. Malnutrition during critical stages of life can lead to irreversible consequences, hindering physical and cognitive development. Breaking the cycle of poverty and food insecurity requires targeted interventions that address the unique needs of these populations.

Climate Change and Agricultural Disruptions:

The increasing frequency and intensity of climate-related events pose a direct threat to agricultural productivity. Droughts, floods, and extreme weather conditions disrupt crop yields and jeopardize food supplies. Implementing sustainable agricultural practices and resilient food systems is crucial for mitigating the impact of climate change on food security.

Globalization and Market Dynamics:

While globalization has expanded access to a variety of foods, it has also introduced challenges such as market volatility and price fluctuations. Vulnerable populations often find themselves at the mercy of these dynamics, struggling to afford a nutritious diet. Implementing policies that regulate markets and support local food production can enhance food security.

Conflict and Displacement:

Regions experiencing conflict and displacement face acute food insecurity challenges. Displacement disrupts access to land, livelihoods, and social support systems, making affected populations highly susceptible to hunger. Humanitarian efforts that provide emergency food aid, support livelihoods, and foster community resilience are critical in such contexts.

Global Collaboration and Sustainable Solutions:

Addressing global food insecurity requires a collaborative approach that spans governments, non-governmental organizations, the private sector, and the global community. Implementing sustainable agricultural practices, investing in infrastructure, and prioritizing education and empowerment initiatives are essential components of long-term solutions.

Empowering Local Communities:

Empowering local communities to build resilient and sustainable food systems is crucial for addressing food insecurity at its roots. Supporting smallholder farmers, promoting agroecological practices, and investing in rural infrastructure can enhance local food production and create self-sufficient communities.

The battle against global food insecurity demands a holistic, global effort that transcends borders and sectors. By addressing root causes, building resilient communities, and fostering sustainable agricultural practices, we can work towards a future where no one is left behind due to a lack of access to food. Through sustained commitment, international cooperation, and a shared vision of a hunger-free world, we can bridge the gap and build a more equitable and food-secure future for all.

Chapter 14

Future Trends in Nutrition

As our understanding of nutrition evolves, so too does the landscape of nutrition science. The future promises innovative discoveries and paradigm shifts that will shape the way we approach food, health, and overall well-being. In this article, we explore the exciting trends in nutrition science that are poised to redefine our understanding of the relationship between diet and human health.

Personalized Nutrition:

The era of one-size-fits-all dietary recommendations is giving way to personalized nutrition. Advances in genetic testing, microbiome research, and artificial intelligence are paving the way for tailored dietary advice based on an individual's unique genetic makeup, gut microbiota, and lifestyle factors. This personalized approach aims to optimize health outcomes and prevent or manage chronic diseases.

Nutrigenomics:

Nutrigenomics, the study of how individual genetic variations influence responses to nutrients, is at the forefront of future nutrition trends. Researchers are unraveling the intricate interplay between genes and dietary components, providing insights into how specific diets can be tailored to mitigate genetic predispositions to certain health conditions.

Microbiome Health:

The gut microbiome, a complex ecosystem of trillions of microorganisms residing in our digestive tract, is emerging as a key player in overall health. Future nutrition science will delve deeper into understanding how the microbiome influences metabolism, immune function, and mental well-being. Probiotics, prebiotics, and personalized nutrition plans will likely play a pivotal role in promoting a healthy gut microbiome.

Functional Foods and Nutraceuticals:

The future of nutrition includes a focus on functional foods and nutraceuticals—foods with additional health benefits beyond basic nutrition. From fortified foods to bioactive compounds extracted from plants, the exploration of functional ingredients is expected to rise. These foods may offer targeted health benefits, ranging from improved cognitive function to enhanced immune support.

Plant-Based and Sustainable Diets:

A shift toward plant-based diets and sustainable eating practices is gaining momentum. Future nutrition trends will likely emphasize the health and environmental benefits of reducing reliance on animal products. Plant-based proteins, alternative meat products, and eco-friendly eating choices will become increasingly prominent in dietary recommendations.

Technology Integration:

The integration of technology into nutrition science is transforming the way we monitor and manage our diets. Mobile apps, wearable devices, and smart kitchen appliances will play a role in tracking nutritional intake, providing real-time feedback, and offering personalized recommendations to support healthier eating habits.

Culinary Medicine:

The convergence of nutrition science and culinary arts is giving rise to culinary medicine—an approach that combines the art of cooking with evidence-based nutrition principles. Medical professionals and chefs collaborate to create nutritious, flavorful meals that align with health recommendations, making healthy eating an enjoyable and accessible part of daily life.

Nutrition for Mental Health:

The link between nutrition and mental health is gaining prominence. Future research is likely to explore how dietary patterns and specific nutrients influence brain function, mood, and mental well-being. Nutritional psychiatry, an emerging field, may provide insights into using nutrition as a therapeutic approach for mental health disorders.

The future of nutrition science is a dynamic landscape, marked by personalized approaches, cutting-edge technologies, and a holistic understanding of the intricate connections between diet and health. As these trends unfold, individuals are empowered to make informed choices that not only nourish their bodies but also contribute to a sustainable and healthier global future. Embracing these evolving trends in nutrition science ensures that we navigate tomorrow's plate with knowledge, purpose, and a commitment to well-being.

Technological Advances in Food Science

As technology continues to advance, the realm of food science is undergoing a revolutionary transformation. From farm to fork, cutting-edge technologies are reshaping the way we produce, process, and consume food. In this article, we explore the latest technological advances in food science that promise to enhance food safety, sustainability, and overall quality, ushering in a new era for the global food industry.

Precision Agriculture:

Precision agriculture leverages technologies such as drones, sensors, and satellite imagery to optimize farming practices. Farmers can monitor crop health, soil conditions, and pest presence in real-time, allowing for precise resource allocation. This data-driven approach enhances crop yields, reduces environmental impact, and ensures more sustainable agricultural practices.

Genetic Editing:

Advances in genetic editing, particularly CRISPR-Cas9 technology, are revolutionizing crop development. Scientists can now modify the genetic makeup of plants to enhance desirable traits, such as resistance to pests, diseases, or environmental stress. This technology holds the potential to create more resilient crops with improved nutritional profiles.

Smart Packaging:

Smart packaging integrates technology to monitor and improve food safety and quality. Innovations include temperature-sensitive labels, freshness indicators, and QR codes that provide consumers with detailed information about the product's journey from production to consumption. These technologies contribute to reducing food waste and ensuring product integrity.

Blockchain for Traceability:

Blockchain technology is being implemented to enhance the traceability of food supply chains. By creating an unalterable digital ledger of each step in the production and distribution process, blockchain ensures transparency and accountability. This not only helps in quickly identifying and addressing food safety issues but also builds trust among consumers.

Vertical Farming and Controlled-Environment Agriculture:

Vertical farming and controlled-environment agriculture utilize indoor farming techniques, including hydroponics and aeroponics, to cultivate crops in vertically stacked layers. These methods optimize resource use, reduce the need for arable land, and enable year-round production. This technology is particularly promising for urban areas with limited space.

3D Printing of Food:

3D printing is making its mark in the food industry, allowing for the creation of intricate and customized food structures. From chocolate sculptures to personalized pasta shapes, this technology offers new possibilities for chefs and food manufacturers. In the future, 3D printing may also contribute to addressing global food security challenges.

Lab-Grown Meat:

Cultured or lab-grown meat is a breakthrough in sustainable protein production. Using cellular agriculture techniques, scientists can grow meat in a controlled environment without the need for traditional livestock farming. This technology has the potential to address environmental concerns associated with conventional meat production.

AI and Machine Learning in Flavor Development:

Artificial intelligence (AI) and machine learning algorithms are being employed to analyze vast datasets and predict flavor profiles. This technology aids food scientists in developing new and innovative flavor combinations, optimizing recipes, and creating personalized taste experiences.

Nutrigenomics and Personalized Nutrition:

Nutrigenomics, the study of how individual genetics influence responses to nutrients, is shaping the field of personalized nutrition. Integrating genetic information with dietary advice enables personalized dietary recommendations tailored to an individual's unique genetic makeup, promoting optimal health outcomes.

The technological advances in food science outlined here represent just the tip of the iceberg in a rapidly evolving field. From revolutionizing agriculture to redefining how we experience flavor, these innovations hold the promise of creating a more sustainable, safe, and personalized food future. Embracing these technologies not only enhances efficiency in the food industry but also contributes to addressing global challenges such as food security, environmental sustainability, and public health. As technology continues to progress, the food science landscape will undoubtedly witness further transformative breakthroughs, shaping the way we nourish ourselves for generations to come.

Shaping the Future of Nutrition Research

Nutrition research stands at the forefront of advancing our understanding of the close relationship between food and health. As technology evolves and interdisciplinary collaborations flourish, the future of nutrition research holds great promise. Following are some of the innovations and perspectives that are shaping the trajectory of nutrition research, paving the way for personalized dietary recommendations, novel interventions, and a deeper understanding of the impact of nutrition on overall well-being.

Omics Technologies:

The integration of omics technologies, including genomics, proteomics, metabolomics, and microbiomics, is transforming nutrition research. Scientists can now analyze vast datasets to unravel the complex interactions between genetics, dietary components, and the gut microbiome. This holistic approach provides insights into individualized responses to nutrients and the underlying mechanisms influencing health outcomes.

Precision Nutrition:

Building on the foundation laid by omics technologies, precision nutrition is emerging as a key focus. The goal is to tailor dietary recommendations to an individual's unique genetic makeup, lifestyle, and health status. Precision nutrition not only considers genetic factors but also incorporates data from wearables, gut microbiome analyses, and other personalized health metrics.

Longitudinal Studies and Big Data:

Longitudinal studies, tracking individuals over extended periods, coupled with big data analytics, offer a comprehensive understanding of the impact of nutrition on health throughout the lifespan. Large-scale datasets enable researchers to identify patterns, correlations, and potential risk factors, providing valuable insights for public health recommendations and interventions.

Interdisciplinary Approaches:

Nutrition research is increasingly benefiting from interdisciplinary collaborations that bridge the gap between different scientific disciplines. Collaborations between nutritionists, geneticists, microbiologists, psychologists, and other experts allow for a more comprehensive understanding of the multifaceted factors influencing dietary behaviors and health outcomes.

Artificial Intelligence and Machine Learning:

Artificial intelligence (AI) and machine learning are revolutionizing data analysis in nutrition research. These technologies can sift through vast amounts of data to identify complex patterns, predict outcomes, and uncover novel associations. In nutrition, AI is being used to analyze dietary patterns, assess nutritional status, and even predict individual responses to specific diets.

Nutrigenetics and Nutrigenomics:

Nutrigenetics explores how individual genetic variations influence responses to nutrients, while nutrigenomics examines the broader impact of nutrition on gene expression. The integration of these fields enables researchers to decipher the genetic basis of nutritional responses, paving the way for targeted dietary interventions based on an individual's genetic profile.

Microbiome Research:

The gut microbiome, a complex ecosystem of microorganisms in the digestive tract, is a burgeoning area of research in nutrition. Understanding the role of the microbiome in nutrient metabolism, immune function, and overall health provides new avenues for developing interventions that support a healthy gut microbiome and, in turn, human health.

Behavioral Nutrition:

Behavioral nutrition investigates the psychological and social factors influencing dietary choices. Insights from behavioral research can inform strategies to promote healthier eating habits, address food preferences, and design interventions that are more likely to be adopted and sustained by individuals.

Public Health Nutrition Interventions:

Future nutrition research is likely to place increased emphasis on developing and evaluating public health interventions. These may include policy recommendations, community-based programs, and educational initiatives aimed at promoting healthier dietary patterns and reducing the burden of diet-related diseases on a population level.

The future of nutrition research is characterized by a dynamic landscape of technological advancements, interdisciplinary collaborations, and a personalized approach to understanding the impact of food on health. As these innovations unfold, they hold the potential to revolutionize dietary recommendations, inform public health policies, and empower individuals to make choices that optimize their well-being. By staying at the forefront of these developments, the field of nutrition research is poised to shape a healthier and more personalized future for individuals and populations alike.

Chapter 15

Regulatory Framework

Regulatory Framework and its Role in Indian and International Market

The nutraceutical industry, encompassing a diverse range of products that bridge the gap between food and pharmaceuticals, has seen remarkable growth worldwide. However, the regulatory landscape governing nutraceuticals varies significantly from country to country.

United States (FDA):

In the United States, the Food and Drug Administration (FDA) oversees the regulation of nutraceuticals. Dietary supplements, a category that includes many nutraceuticals, fall under the Dietary Supplement Health and Education Act (DSHEA). This legislation outlines specific requirements for labeling, safety, and good manufacturing practices. Nutraceutical manufacturers must ensure that their products meet these standards, and the FDA has the authority to take action against unsafe or misbranded products.

European Union (EFSA):

The European Union (EU) regulates nutraceuticals through the European Food Safety Authority (EFSA). The EU follows a centralized approach, requiring pre-market authorization for health claims associated with nutraceutical products. The European Commission maintains a list of approved health claims based on scientific evidence. Nutraceutical manufacturers must adhere to these regulations to market their products within the EU.

Canada (Health Canada):

In Canada, the regulation of nutraceuticals falls under the purview of Health Canada. The Natural Health Products Regulations govern the licensing, labeling, and safety of nutraceuticals. Health claims must be supported by scientific evidence, and manufacturers must obtain a product license before marketing. This regulatory framework aims to ensure the safety and efficacy of nutraceuticals for Canadian consumers.

Japan (FOSHU):

Japan has a unique regulatory framework for nutraceuticals known as Foods for Specified Health Uses (FOSHU). The system, overseen by the Ministry of Health, Labour and Welfare (MHLW), requires scientific evidence to support health claims associated with nutraceuticals. Products meeting FOSHU criteria receive official approval and can make specific health claims on their labels.

India (FSSAI):

In India, the Food Safety and Standards Authority of India (FSSAI) regulates nutraceuticals under the Food Safety and Standards (Health Supplements, Nutraceuticals, Food for Special Dietary Use, Food for Special Medical Purpose,

Functional Food, and Novel Food) Regulations. These regulations provide a framework for the approval, labeling, and safety standards for nutraceuticals in the Indian market.

Australia and New Zealand (FSANZ):

The regulation of nutraceuticals in Australia and New Zealand is overseen by Food Standards Australia New Zealand (FSANZ). The Australia New Zealand Food Standards Code sets out requirements for labeling, safety, and health claims. Nutraceutical manufacturers must ensure compliance with these standards to market their products in this region.

China (CFDA):

China regulates nutraceuticals through the China Food and Drug Administration (CFDA). Nutraceuticals are classified as health foods, and manufacturers must obtain approval from the CFDA before marketing. The regulations include requirements for safety, efficacy, and labeling of health foods, ensuring consumer protection.

Brazil (ANVISA):

In Brazil, the National Health Surveillance Agency (ANVISA) oversees the regulation of nutraceuticals. The regulatory framework includes specific rules for the registration, labeling, and safety of dietary supplements and other nutraceutical products. Manufacturers must comply with these regulations to market their products in Brazil.

The regulatory landscape for nutraceuticals is complex and varies considerably across different countries. As the nutraceutical industry continues to grow, harmonizing global regulations becomes an essential consideration to ensure consumer safety, facilitate international trade, and promote innovation in this dynamic sector. Navigating these diverse regulatory frameworks requires diligence from manufacturers and a nuanced understanding of the specific requirements in each market.

FSSAI in India: Safeguarding Food Safety and Nutrition

The Food Safety and Standards Authority of India (FSSAI) plays a pivotal role in ensuring the safety and quality of food products consumed by millions of people across the country. Established to regulate and streamline food-related laws in India, FSSAI has emerged as a crucial authority that governs various aspects of the food industry. In this article, we delve into the role of FSSAI in India, its functions, and its impact on the nation's food safety and nutrition landscape.

Formation of FSSAI:

Established in 2006 under the Food Safety and Standards Act, FSSAI operates as an autonomous body under the Ministry of Health and Family Welfare, Government of India. The primary objective is to consolidate and streamline various food laws, setting standards to ensure the availability of safe and wholesome food for consumption.

Key Functions of FSSAI:

Setting Standards:

One of FSSAI's fundamental functions is to set standards for food products and ingredients. These standards encompass a wide range of factors, including permissible additives, maximum residue limits for pesticides, and guidelines for labeling and packaging. These standards are aimed at ensuring the safety and quality of food products available in the Indian market.

Licensing and Registration:

FSSAI is responsible for licensing and registration of food businesses operating in India. This includes manufacturers, distributors, retailers, and even importers of food products. By implementing a comprehensive licensing system, FSSAI aims to monitor and regulate food businesses, ensuring compliance with safety standards.

Food Safety Surveillance:

FSSAI conducts rigorous surveillance to monitor and assess the safety of food products in the market. This involves regular inspections, sampling, and testing of food items to identify and address potential risks. Through its surveillance efforts, FSSAI aims to prevent the distribution and sale of unsafe or adulterated food products.

Promoting Food Safety Education:

FSSAI actively engages in promoting food safety awareness and education. The authority works to empower consumers, food businesses, and various stakeholders with information on safe food practices. This includes campaigns, workshops, and collaborations to enhance food safety knowledge across the country.

Regulating Advertisements and Claims:

FSSAI regulates advertisements and claims made by food businesses to ensure they are accurate and comply with established standards. This helps in preventing misleading information and false claims about the nutritional content and health benefits of food products.

Impact on Food Safety and Nutrition:

Ensuring Safe Food Supply: FSSAI's stringent standards and regulations contribute significantly to ensuring the safety of the food supply chain in India. By setting and enforcing standards, the authority plays a crucial role in preventing the distribution of substandard or adulterated food products.

Building Consumer Confidence: FSSAI's activities, including regular inspections, testing, and surveillance, help build consumer confidence in the safety and quality of the food they consume. A robust regulatory framework ensures that consumers can make informed choices, knowing that the food products meet established safety standards.

Preventing Foodborne Illnesses: FSSAI's focus on surveillance and proactive measures aids in preventing foodborne illnesses. By identifying and addressing potential risks early in the food supply chain, the authority contributes to reducing the incidence of foodborne diseases and protecting public health.

Facilitating Trade and Industry Growth: FSSAI's licensing and registration system provides a structured framework for food businesses, facilitating fair trade practices and industry growth. This regulatory oversight ensures that businesses comply with safety standards, fostering a competitive and transparent marketplace.

FSSAI's role in India is pivotal to ensuring that the nation's food supply is safe, wholesome, and adheres to established standards. By regulating various aspects of the food industry, from setting standards to monitoring food businesses and promoting consumer awareness, FSSAI plays a crucial role in safeguarding public health and nutrition. As India continues to evolve as a major player in the global food market, FSSAI's commitment to food safety and quality will remain paramount in shaping the nation's food landscape.

Chapter 16

Conclusion

The Ongoing Journey Towards Optimal Nutrition

As we reach the final chapters of this exploration into the vast realm of nutrition, it becomes evident that the journey towards optimal well-being is an ongoing odyssey, a perpetual quest for nourishment that extends beyond the pages of this book. Throughout our exploration, we have unearthed the intricacies of dietary patterns, dissected the science behind superfoods, and delved into the dynamic relationship between nutrition and health. As we conclude, let us reflect on the key takeaways and the roadmap ahead in the ongoing journey towards optimal nutrition.

Understanding the Nuances:

The journey towards optimal nutrition requires an understanding of the nuanced interplay between dietary choices, lifestyle, genetics, and the environment. It is a journey that transcends simplistic notions of good or bad foods, acknowledging the unique needs of individuals and recognizing that optimal nutrition is a personalized pursuit.

Balancing Act:

Achieving optimal nutrition is akin to striking a delicate balance on the nutritional tightrope. It involves a judicious mix of macronutrients, micronutrients, and hydration, coupled with an awareness of portion sizes and the importance of variety in dietary choices. Striking this balance is an ongoing process that evolves with changing circumstances and individual needs.

The Power of Whole Foods:

Throughout our exploration, the recurring theme has been the undeniable power of whole, unprocessed foods. From vibrant fruits and vegetables to nutrient-dense grains and proteins, whole foods form the bedrock of optimal nutrition. Embracing a predominantly plant-based, whole-food diet is a cornerstone of this ongoing journey.

Mindful Eating:

Mindful eating invites us to savor each bite, paying attention to the flavors, textures, and sensations that accompany the act of nourishing our bodies. In a world inundated with fast-paced lifestyles, the practice of mindful eating provides a compass for the ongoing journey, fostering a deeper connection with the food we consume.

Adaptability and Flexibility:

The journey towards optimal nutrition demands adaptability and flexibility. Recognizing that individual needs change over time, influenced by age, activity levels, and life circumstances, empowers us to adjust our nutritional approach accordingly. This ongoing process of adaptation ensures that our dietary choices remain attuned to the ever-changing tapestry of our lives.

Lifelong Learning:

The field of nutrition is dynamic, with research continually unveiling new insights. Embracing a spirit of lifelong learning is essential in navigating the ongoing journey towards optimal nutrition. Staying informed about emerging research, nutritional trends, and evolving dietary guidelines ensures that our choices align with the latest evidence-based recommendations.

As we bring this chapter to a close, it is essential to acknowledge that the journey towards optimal nutrition is not a destination but a perpetual expedition. It is a journey marked by self-discovery, resilience, and an unwavering commitment to health and well-being. The pages of this book are but a guide, a compass pointing towards a future where individuals are empowered to make informed choices, and where communities prioritize the significance of nutritional literacy.

In the ongoing quest for optimal nutrition, each meal becomes an opportunity, each food choice a step forward, and each day a chance to nourish the body and nurture well-being. Let this book be a beacon, illuminating the path towards a future where the journey towards optimal nutrition is embraced with curiosity, mindfulness, and a profound appreciation for the remarkable relationship between what we eat and how we live. May this journey be as enriching and nourishing as the food that fuels it. Bon voyage on your ongoing quest towards nutritional nirvana.